NUTRITIONAL HEALERS

How to Eat Your Way to Better Health

Other Books by the Author

Helping Your Health with Enzymes
Natural Hormones: The Secret of Youthful Health
The Miracle of Organic Vitamins for Better Health
Slimfasting—The Quick "Pounds Off" Way to Youthful Slimness
Healing and Revitalizing Your Vital Organs
Encyclopedia of Power Foods for Health and Longer Life
Inner Cleansing—Free Yourself from
  Joint-Muscle-Artery-Circulation Sludge
Eat Away Illness: How to Age-Proof Your Body with Antioxidant Foods

NUTRITIONAL HEALERS

How to Eat Your Way to Better Health

Carlson Wade

Parker Publishing Company, Inc.
West Nyack, N.Y.

© 1987 *by*

PARKER PUBLISHING COMPANY, INC.

West Nyack, N.Y.

10 9 8 7 6 5 4 3 2 1
10 9 8 7 6 5 4 3 2 1

This book is a reference work based on research by
the author. The opinions expressed herein are not
necessary those of or endorsed by the publisher. The
directions stated in this book are in no way to be
considered as a substitute for consultation with a duly
licensed doctor.

DEDICATION

To a Longer and Healthier Life...
Filled with Youthful Happiness

Library of Congress Cataloging-in-Publication Data

Wade, Carlson.
  Nutritional healers.

  Includes index.
  1. Diet therapy. 2. Nutrition. I. Title.
  [DNLM: 1. Diet Therapy—popular works. 2. Nutrition—
popular works. WB 400 W119n]
  RM216.W29 1987   613.2   87-1373

ISBN 0-13-627233-9

ISBN 0-13-627225-8 PBK

Printed in the United States of America

Foreword by a Medical Doctor

In my medical practice, I see many health-conscious people who are concerned about the use of drugs for such conditions as arthritis, high blood pressure, cancer, cardiovascular disorders, allergies, and gastrointestinal problems. My patients want to feel good and look youthful while healing many common and uncommon disorders. They frequently ask if there is an alternative route to possibly addictive drugs and surgery. Happily, I am able to recommend highly the use of nutritional therapy as researched by the highly respected medical reporter, Carlson Wade.

This new guide to total healing of body and mind with the use of nutrition is designed for the complete person. The programs show you how to use everyday foods and nutrients to allow your body to initiate healing from within. These programs may be considered "natural medicines" because they work so effectively, but unlike chemotherapeutic drugs, they are free of side effects. Neither are they habit forming. They work on an entirely new set of principles of healing as revealed by Carlson Wade, namely, an inner transformation. Nutritional healers promote internal rejuvenation and stimulation of the immune system to overcome stubborn conditions.

This book is on the latest scientific findings about the effective treatment of many illnesses with the use of everyday foods. It takes you by the hand and guides you through the inner workings and mechanisms of a specific condition, then it gives you highly workable nutritional programs you can use in the privacy of your own home as a means of fast and effective healing. Often, the programs can give you lifetime freedom from problems you thought were hopeless!

With simple, easy-to-follow programs, you have a personalized nutritional healing prescription to help you to overcome debilitative conditions and boost the strength of your immune system to enjoy total health in the many years ahead. And thanks to the powerful and workable nutritional therapies presented by Carlson Wade, you will look better and feel better. This book should be in *everyone's* hands. It is the key to total rejuvenation and healing with the use of corrective foods. You will live longer and much, much better with Carlson Wade's highly recommended book. It works!

H. W. Holderby, M.D.

What This Book Will Do for You

A set of eight major diseases take 160 lives an hour. In the struggle for survival against killer illnesses, we see more than 4,000 Americans die every single day. The modern-day plagues—heart trouble, cancer, cerebrovascular disease, lung problems, respiratory disorders, diabetes, liver troubles, kidney failure—have proved to be among the most ruthless killers in our country. Even with high-tech science and computerized medicine, the fatalities still mount.

Additionally, there are crippling ailments that include blood pressure trouble, excess fatty accumulation, arthritis, allergies, stress, osteoporosis, the fear of memory loss via Alzheimer's disease, and nagging digestive disorders such as painful ulcers or irritating heartburn. We are troubled with obesity as well as everyday headache, muscle, or stress pain. The greatest problem is that of unwarranted premature old age.

In researching for therapies that would ease distress, promote healing, and give hope for a cure, I came across a treasure of nutritional therapies. The comparatively young science of using foods as medicine is being utilized and recognized by leading medical experts as a means of boosting the body's own immune system. The reaction is to fight illness from within and invigorate the body so it can recuperate and cast out infectious threats.

Gathering these latest nutritional doctrines in a book became a dedicated goal in my profession as a medical researcher and reporter. Not only did I criss-cross the country in search of answers to nutritional healing questions, but I talked to countless people, including experts in the field of health and nutrition. The purpose was to offer an alternative to drugs for more than the nation's most deadly killer diseases, that is, for just about any common disorder. Gradually, the book began to take shape as the nutritional therapies were outlined just as they had been used to snatch many from fatality or lifelong disability.

This book is a compendium of the best medical minds in the field of nutritional healing from all parts of the country. The programs use *no* drugs, *no* confinement, *no* unusual or costly devices. Many of the ingredients are in your pantry right now, or else they are available at your nearby food outlet. Many of the healers are so simple, they can be used in a matter of moments. Healing is just as swift, according to the researchers.

Why is nutrition so vital as a healing method? We currently spend some $2 billion a year searching for cures but 100 times more on treatments. It costs us upwards of $200 billion annually, or about $1,000 for every man, woman, and child in the country, for sick leave, doctors, hospitals, drugs, and surgery to treat these chronic killers. After years of investigation, it has been found that there are many opportunities to prevent such illnesses, and even more nutritional programs to help bring about effective treatment. The cost would be a fraction of spiralling hospitalization or lifetime drug taking. The book you now hold in your hands is a breakthrough in the search for alternatives to costly, painful, and often fatal consequences of conventional chemotherapy and surgery.

If you or anyone you know is troubled with any of the eight major diseases of the 1980s, this book is for you. For problems of stress, stiffness, poor memory, gastritis, heartburn, muscle or neurological pains of any sort, hypoglycemia, prostate trouble, menstrual syndrome, poor blood health, and premature aging, this book will share the findings of top nutritional and medical sciences the world over.

The very new science of the immune system is also discussed with a variety of newly discovered nutritional methods to help boost resistance against a variety of assaults on your mental and physical heatlh.

The use of just one program may well save a life...of someone you know, or even your own!

You can win the battle against major and minor illnesses with the use of nutritional therapy. This book will show you how to reverse the tide of aging and tap the wells of healing with drugless methods. Thanks to this new research, it is possible for you to protect yourself against killing or crippling ailments—become totally healed and enjoy the best that is to come, with the use of nutritional healers.

Carlson Wade

Contents

How to Ease and Erase Arthritis Distress with Healing Foods

Arthritis? Why me?"

This question is asked when an apparently healthy person is told that arthritis has taken hold and may worsen as the years go on. The traditional answer is either "heredity" or else "trauma" of one sort or another.

"Can my arthritis be cured?"

It is only natural for the patient to want to live *without* arthritis. This question shows a desire to want to heal and erase this health threat. The usual answer is that arthritis has no cure and that the most that can be done is to submit to various types of drug therapy and medication. It may be an occasional drug. It usually means a lifetime of chemotherapy. There is little hope beyond being drugged so that the pain of arthritis is not felt. But it increases in silent or drugged intensity because medications are directed at *symptoms,* not at the *causes* of arthritis. Under this regimen, *arthritis may well be forever.*

With the newer knowledge of nutritional science, you do have an alternative. You can find relief from pain and even healing of this threatening crippler with the use of newly discovered nutritional therapy. A dietary approach can be aimed at correcting the *cause* of this distress; once this *metabolic error* has been corrected, the symptoms subside and you may look forward to a life that is free of arthritis.

Before You Begin

There are different nutritional therapies. You may respond better to one program than to another. Since each person is different, each one will have a different response to the dietary program. You need to pursue the different therapies until you find one that offers you the relief you seek. When you feel the long-term control of symptoms because of one or more nutritional therapies, then you will assume that you are on the right track and look ahead to freedom from arthritis. It is up to you, with the help of your medical nutritionist, to find the proper program for your specific needs.

Arthritis: Something You Ate...
Or Didn't Eat?

Is Arthritis a Food Allergy?

Something you ate may trigger arthritis flare-up. There are certain foods that upset the metabolic balance and can be blamed for causing an allergic reaction with the symptoms of arthritis! In particular, scientists have found that one group of foods, the *nightshade plant group*, can cause painful arthritic flare-ups, even if taken in small amounts. Eliminate these foods, and you may be able to eliminate arthritis.

What Are the Nightshade Foods?

These include four basic everyday foods: *white potato, tomato, eggplant,* and *red pepper.* They may be healthfully, nutritious foods for many people, but for others, they tend to trigger an allergic reaction that erupts as arthritis flare-up. By absolutely avoiding these four foods, you may well be able to turn the tide and bolster resistance to arthritis distress.

The Toxic Trigger in Nightshade Foods. Nightshade foods contain an ingredient identified as *solanine,* a bitter, toxic, crystalline alkaloid that causes a metabolic shock to trigger arthritic distress. It is a saponic like glycoalkaloid that irritates by destroying red blood cells to cause a general breakdown.

Solanine is an inhibitor of cholinesterase, an enzyme that provides agility of muscle movements. This toxic trigger can destroy the important enzyme and make you vulnerable to stiffness, sluggish muscle movements, painful spasms. If you are troubled with arthritis, check your nutritional program. If you eliminate the four foods of the nightshade family, you may well free your body from the destructive solanine toxic trigger and enjoy freedom from arthritis!

ERASES "HOPELESS" ARTHRITIS IN NINE DAYS WITH SIMPLE DIET CHANGE

Martha A. was so troubled with cripplinglike rheumatoid arthritis she could hardly hold a spoon in her pain-wracked hand. Housework was agonizing. There was no relief from stubborn pains, especially in the morning. She was told to "live with it" because chemotherapy offered partial help but could not heal arthritis. But Martha A. was determined to find an alternative or natural therapy for her condition.

A medical nutritionist prepared a complete dietary and physical profile for her. She was told to self-test by eliminating the four nightshade plants from her diet. Here response would be monitored to see if her arthritis was due to an allergic reaction to these solanine-containing foods. Martha A. followed this simple diet change. No white potato, no tomato, no eggplant, no red pepper in any form. Results? Within four days, her hands and fingers felt more flexible. In seven days, she could move around the house and grounds with youthful agility. By the ninth day, she was pronounced "free" from the formerly "hopeless" arthritis. Martha A. became so energetic by this nutritional therapy, she soon took on a full-time job because she liked being active. It was her way of celebrating her freedom from arthritis!

Be Alert to "Hidden" Forms of Nightshade Foods. These four "no-no" foods that may be responsible for allergic reactions of arthritis are found in packaged products. You may be eating them in the form of starch, filler, flavoring, spices, coloring, vegetables, without knowing it. Be sure to *read labels* of any packaged or processed foods. Be aware of seemingly innocent listings such as "starch" or "fillers" which are often made of these nightshade foods.

Eating Out?

Restaurant eating calls for planning. Salads, soups, stews, casseroles, baked foods, meat or vegetable pies, even sandwiches may have one or more of these four "no-no" foods, either as part of the original recipe or adding during preparation. Even a small portion could cause an arthritis flare-up, *if* you are allergic to these foods. Be prepared *before* you eat out to protect yourself.

Whole Foods Are Safe Foods. When eating out, select whole foods that will be free of these nightshades. *Examples:* consider a lean cut of meat, slice of seafood, dairy-based entrée, steamed fresh or raw vegetables, and freshly prepared legumes. *Careful:* beware of stews, burgers, and canned or frozen foods. You will be less likely to have an arthritic-allergic attack due to the solanine toxic trigger if you stick to whole foods.

Yes, the nightshades are nutritious foods. For many people, they can build health without arthritic or other allergic reactions. But for others, they can cause distress. If you belong to this latter group, try a simple elimination diet. The vitamins, minerals, and enzymes found in these "no-no" foods are easily obtainable in most other fresh fruits, vegetables, and whole grains. This easy diet change may well help you enjoy arthritis-free health.

Arthritis: The Current Problem

More than 36 million Americans have some form of arthritis. Each year, 1 million people will learn they have some form of this threat. About 250,000 children have juvenile arthritis. It is estimated that arthritis costs our country over $13 billion yearly in hospitalization, physician visits, drugs, nursing home care, lost wages and homemaker services, and earnings lost because of premature death.

We cannot put a dollar figure on the emotional and physical effects of living with this chronic and serious disease. Nor can we include many other costs such as those spent on disability payments to people whose arthritis has left them unable to work for a living. The problem knows no limits.

What Is Arthritis?

The word arthritis literally means "joint inflammation." That is, *arth* means "joint" and *itis* means "inflammation." It is not a single disease, but rather a symptom that can occur in more than 100 acute and chronic conditions. Two basic forms of arthritis appear to respond to nutritional correction:

Osteoarthritis. Considered the "most common form," it involves the breakdown of cartilage and other joint tissues. It causes little or no inflammation and does not affect the whole body. Probably every person over age 60 has it to some degree, but only a few have it badly enough to notice any symptoms. These usually begin slowly. One or two joints may ache or feel mildly sore, especially with movement. There may be some constant nagging pain. Usually, symptoms are their worst after the joints have been overused or have remained still for a long period. While osteoarthritis can occur in any joint, those most commonly affected are the fingers, hips, knees, and spine.

Rheumatoid Arthritis. An inflammation of the joint membrane. If neglected, outgrowths of the inflamed tissue may invade and damage the cartilage in the synovial (joint-lining) joints. This injury may change the shape of the joints, causing them to become deformed. Early in the condition, most people feel tired, sore, achy, and stiff. The joints stiffen, then swell, and become tender, later making full motion difficult and painful. The symptoms are often worst in the morning and after long periods of sitting or lying still. The knees, hands, and feet are commonly involved. Often, the joints on both sides of the body are affected. That is, both feet, or both hips are involved. In some people (about one out of six) the condition becomes severe, causing aches, pains, and badly affected joints. For example, the fingers may become crooked and deformed; movement is painful and difficult.

Juvenile Arthritis

Not exclusively an "old person's condition," we have identified several forms of juvenile arthritis. The condition may appear any time after birth, often before the age of 7. In most cases, it first affects a child's knees. The effects can change from day to day, even from morning to afternoon.

Affected children may experience skin rash, fever, inflammation of the eyes, slowed growth, swelling of lymph nodes, fatigue, and swelling and pain in the muscles and joints. Either a few or many joints may be afflicted. Some youngsters recover completely. Others may be troubled with it during their adult lives.

With the use of corrective nutritional therapy and an improved lifestyle, a youngster can be given hope for a lifetime that will be free of arthritis.

A Doctor's Nutritional Therapy for Healing Arthritis[1]

For several decades, an arthritis medical clinic has used nutritional therapy as part of a total body healing program to treat over tens of

---

[1]Robert Bingham, M.D., Desert Hot Springs Medical Clinic, Calif., press release, 1984.

thousands of arthritics with much success. Founder–medical director, Robert Bingham, M.D., a certified member of the American Board of Orthopedic Surgery and Fellow of the American Academy of Orthopedic Surgery, explains that by making changes in the diet, taking prescribed amounts of vitamins and minerals, there is hope to block rheumatoid arthritis and reverse degenerative forms of this disease.

The Diet Connection in Arthritis

Dr. Bingham explains, "Nutritional science teaches us (1) how crucial the internal environment of our body cells and tissues is; (2) that the nutrition we receive in food may shape and build our entire lives; and (3) all kinds of diseases and malformations such as arthritis are rooted in poor internal environment from dietary deficiencies."

He adds: "Medicines and drugs interfere with metabolism, but nutrients make metabolism possible. They are the raw materials from which metabolic machinery is built. Life cannot exist without them.

"The intricate balance of nutrients in the body involves the interrelationships among forty or more such substances. *An extremely poor nutritional balance may result in deficiency diseases;* a poor or mediocre balance yields at best sub-optimal health and vigor.

"Nutrition has been in lethargy for too long. It needs to be taken seriously by biochemists, medical scientists, medical educators, and family physicians.

"Vast human betterment—including substantial relief from coronary heart disease, birth defects, arthritis, mental disease, alcoholism, dental disease, muscular dystrophy, multiple sclerosis, cataracts, glaucoma, cancer, and many other diseases—must await the day when nutrition comes alive and reaches out to new horizons."

The Step-by-Step Nutritional Therapy for Arthritis

At his world-famous arthritis clinic, Dr. Bingham offers a program that, he says, could also be followed to a lesser degree at home to help reverse the tide of this condition. Here is this step-by-step nutritional therapy plan that has helped tens of thousands free themselves from arthritis.

1. Avoid all refined flour products, refined sugar, or sweets.

2. Daily, increase well-absorbed calcium to 6 oyster shell tablets a day. For osteoarthritis, Dr. Bingham recommends 1,000 units daily of vitamin D from a natural source such as halibut liver oil. Take this with 25,000 units daily of vitamin A. *Note:* This combination is for the treatment phase. For prevention, the doctor suggests half this amount.

3. Increase water consumption to 8 or more glasses a day.

4. Put yourself on a high-protein diet.

5. Eat only fresh, raw, natural fruits and vegetables—use a blender or grinder to prepare as needed. Cook only if absolutely necessary.

6. Eliminate tobacco, alcohol, refined carbohydrates, and saturated fats.

7. If overweight, lose the excess poundage. But be careful to get adequate protein from skim milk dairy products, lean poultry, fish, and lean meats as well as nuts, whole grains, and seeds. A blender and a grinder are beneficial in maximizing the use of such fresh, natural foods, says the doctor.

8. Ask your medical nutritionist for specific nutritional potencies for your personal condition. Generally, the arthritic is in need of additional vitamin B-complex, vitamin C, vitamin D, and iron. Drugs taken for arthritis tend to deplete these nutrients, compounding the problem.

9. Drink fresh milk as it offers a number of important vitamins and minerals, especially calcium, that helps to ease arthritis distress. "Certified raw milk, if available, is highly recommended," says Dr. Bingham. "It is higher in enzymes, hormone growth factors, protein, available minerals and fats and natural vitamins than pasteurized milk. It is especially valuable for those with a tendency to arthritis. Buttermilk has the same protein value as whole milk and contains no more fat than skim milk. Certified raw milk has the Wulzen factor or an antistiffness benefit that is important for easing arthritis distress."

10. Keep yourself physically active so that nutrients can perform their healing therapy. Many people are deficient in bone and muscle protein, bone calcium, and good joint cartilage, with excessive fat deposits in the tissue, body organs, and the arteries. Activity helps to put nutrients to active use in correcting arthritis distress.

With the assistance of a medical nutritionist, this 10-step program, as prescribed by Dr. Bingham at his arthritis clinic, may help to reverse the tide of this insidious and often-crippling disease.

Dr. Bingham asserts that not only is arthritis preventable with nutritional therapy, but it can be curable, too.

How to "Oil" Your Joints and Ease Arthritic Pain

For many arthritics, the ingestion of fish liver oil eases arthritic pain. What began as a folk remedy is now being seen as possibly having a biochemical basis. In studies, it was found that 1 or 2 tablespoons of cod liver oil, taken with milk at bedtime, was able to help ease joint stiffness and erase much arthritic pain.

"Secret" of Cod Liver Oil as Nutritional Therapy

Cod liver and most fish oils are prime sources of essential fatty acids such as linoleic and linolenic acids. These nutrients cause the outpouring of prostaglandins; these are potent hormonelike substances that are able to help block pain receptors, especially in the joints. The oil acts as a spark plug to promote the release of the important prostaglandins that will help to soothe the spasms of joint pain. This is the "secret" of any effectiveness noted from taking fish liver oil.

Simple Nutritional Therapy: About two hours before bedtime, take 2 tablespoons of fish liver oil with milk for easier digestion. You may be able to sleep better and awaken with less of the morning stiffness that is the curse of so many arthritics.

Instead of Aspirin, Try a Nutritional Pain Killer: Phenylalanine

If you are cautious about using chemicals to mask arthritis pain, you will want to use a nutritional alternative. It is a simple amino acid: *phenylalanine.*

What Is It?

Phenylalanine is one of the essential amino acids your body cannot make but must be obtained from your diet or a supplement. It does not exactly kill pain. Instead, it protects your body's own source of pain relief—*endorphins* (Greek for "the morphine within"). These are morphinelike substances produced by your body that block pain signals moving through your nervous system.

During the natural process of digestion, there is some destruction of these endorphins. You become more vulnerable to arthritic and other pains. You need to shield and protect these pain-killing endorphins. You can do it with *phenylalanine,* which is considered a *natural aspirin.*

Eases Pain, Cools Inflammation

This amino acid works speedily to guard the life span and effectiveness of the small endorphins, or enkephalins, which will ease your pain and cool the painful inflammation of arthritis.

More Benefits from "Nutritional Aspirin"

Phenylalanine is not a drug, but it performs like chemicalized aspirin *without* side effects. It is nonaddictive, nontoxic. It acts as a moodlifter. It relieves the depression that often accompanies arthritic suffering. This "nutritional aspirin" has the unique ability to block certain antagonists in the central nervous system from degrading (breaking down) pain-killing endorphins and enkephalins and allows them to act as natural and potent analgesics. It may well be the best "nutritional aspirin" available for relief of arthritis and other painful disorders.

How Much to Take?

A general rule of thumb calls for taking 375 milligrams with your breakfast, another 375 milligrams with your noonday meal, and a third 375 milligrams with your evening meal. Your nutritional health practitioner can recommend specific dosages for your needs.

Caution: Phenylalanine should *not* be taken by pregnant or lactating women or anyone who has the genetic condition of phenyketonuria (PKU) because these people cannot metabolize the nutrient normally. This also applies to those on a phenylalanine-restricted diet. Neither should it be given to children under the age of 14, except under prescribed dosages by the consulting health practitioner.

Where to Find This Nutritional Aspirin

Here are some food sources for phenylalanine and their potencies (Chart 1-1).

Chart 1-1: PHENYLALANINE CONTENT OF EVERYDAY FOODS

	Serving Size	Milligrams of Phenylalanine
Whole milk,	3½ ounces	170
Dried, nonfat milk	3½ ounces	1,724
Cheddar cheese	3½ ounces	1,244
Egg	1 large	739
Beef, chuck	3½ ounces	765
Chicken, fryer	3½ ounces	811
Turkey	3½ ounces	960
Codfish, fresh	3½ ounces	612
Haddock, fresh	3½ ounces	676
Halibut, fresh	3½ ounces	690
Salmon, Pacific, fresh	3½ ounces	646
Peanuts	3½ ounces	1,557
Peanut butter	3½ ounces	1,510
Pecans	3½ ounces	564
Walnuts	3½ ounces	767
Oatmeal, rolled oats	3½ ounces	758
Rice	3½ ounces	382
Farina	3½ ounces	579
Macaroni, spaghetti	3½ ounces	669
Shredded wheat	3½ ounces	755
Beans, lima	3½ ounces	197

Your Pain-Fighting Food Plan:

You can easily plan your daily menu to include just a few (or even one) of the preceding high-phenylalanine–containing foods. This will release a good supply of this valuable amino acid that will protect your endorphins and thereby help your body to unleash them to ease pain and elevate your mood.

PAIN FREE IN SIX DAYS

John R. developed arthritis in his knees five years ago. Not too painful at first, he took aspirin occasionally. Then the arthritis spread to his shoulders, hands, and left elbow. He took more aspirin and prescribed codeine, but these drugs made him feel sick, even if they did soothe the pain. Then he was advised by a physiotherapist to try phenylalanine supplements. He took about a total of 1,000 milligrams a day, in three divided doses. He also began to include foods high in this amino acid. Almost at once, the painful swelling subsided. Within six days, his knees, shoulders, hands, and arms were free of swelling and pain. He discontinued the supplement but continued the food sources of this amino acid. He gave up aspirin and drugs, too. He was soon free of arthritis pain, thanks to the soothing benefits of phenylalanine, which he calls his "food aspirin."

The Doctor Prescribes a Nutritional Therapy Program for Arthritics[2]

A noted physician, Leo V. Roy, M.D., of Toronto, Canada, has found that when arthritics follow a total nutritional therapy program, there is much hope for relief of symptoms and eventual elimination of this condition. Dr. Roy offers this total program to his patients which can be followed at home.

Basic Therapy:

Eat as many fresh raw fruits and vegetables as possible. Chew thoroughly so that saliva is mixed with foods and better utilized. Eat slowly. Avoid large quantities.

Food Program

1. *Proteins:* Every meal should contain a protein. One-fourth of daily food intake should be protein. Best sources: fish, nuts, cheese, eggs, raw certified milk.
2. *Meats:* Use internal organs, rich in vitamins and minerals. Avoid all canned and processed foods. Poultry, lamb, steak are good.
3. *Dairy products:* Eat all cheeses, natural and fermented; yogurt and natural buttermilk.
4. *Raw vegetables:* All are recommended, especially celery, cucumbers, and carrots. Make salads using oils for dressing.
5. *Cooked vegetables:* Baked potatoes and brown rice are nutritious. Use raw bean sprouts and other sprouts. Do *not* overcook any vegetable. Steam, bake, broil, or use as little water as possible.
6. *Fruits:* All are recommended, especially apples, grapes, bananas, or local varieties.

[2]Leo V. Roy, M.D., press release, 1985.

7. *Juices:* Drink freshly-squeezed or bottled grape juice, no sugar added. No tomatoes. No citrus fruits except as flavoring. Maximum of 1 teaspoon lemon juice for salad dressing.

8. *Cereals:* Try the fresh-ground combination—wheat, rye, sesame seed, flax, and millet. Do not boil. Soak 15 to 20 minutes in hot water over a double boiler, or soak overnight and warm. Raw sunflower seeds, raisins, or shredded coconut may be added before eating.

9. *Bread:* Use sparingly and only stone-ground fresh whole wheat or rye.

10. *Soups:* Bouillon or consommé is allowed.

11. *Acid drink:* Where there is insufficient acid or where there are calcium deposits, use 1 tablespoon apple cider vinegar to 1 glass of water (with or without honey, 1 teaspoon) at least twice daily.

12. *Oils:* Consider especially sesame, safflower, and sunflower oil and all seeds and raw nuts.

Avoid all the following:

Tea	Commercial cereals	All hydrogenated (hardened) fats
Coffee	Processed foods	Roasted nuts
Alcohol	Canned meats	Stale nuts
Canned foods	White flour	Stale wheat germ
Stale foods	White sugar	Stale wheat germ oil

Avoid overcooked and reheated foods, jams, jellies, syrups, ice cream, soft drinks, and tobacco; avoid all chemicals added to your food such as sweeteners, emulsifiers, thickeners, and fluoridated water. *Read your labels carefully.*

The therapeutic benefits of this program lie in its ability to help uproot and cast out corrosive or irritating waste products that could be at the root of the arthritic disturbance. It calls for a total nutritional cleansing, which is believed to be the key to healing of arthritis upset.

The preceding program of nutritional therapy has reportedly helped countless arthritic victims find relief from their disorder. You, too, may be able to reverse or, at least, halt the ravages of arthritis with such a program. The sooner you begin, the sooner you may see (and feel) the benefits.

Arthritis may be traced to something you should eat, and other things you should not eat. With these nutritional therapies, you may well be able to learn how to live *without* your so-called "hopeless" arthritis.

HIGHLIGHTS

1. You have an alternative to drugs in finding relief and escape from arthritis in the form of nutritional therapy.
2. Is your arthritis due to an allergic reaction? Eliminate the four "no-no" nightshade foods, and you may well eliminate your arthritis.
3. Martha A. was able to erase her "hopeless" arthritis in nine days with a simple nutritional adjustment.
4. Become familiar with the different forms of arthritis and their causes to help you understand how to cope with this condition.
5. A California doctor has healed thousands of arthritic patients with a nutritional therapy program that is outlined for home use.
6. Fish liver oils may hold the key to pain relief.
7. John R. became pain free in six days with the use of a common nutritional pain killer.
8. A Canadian physician has a nutritional therapy program that helps to relieve symptoms and offers hope for elimination of arthritis. The program can easily be followed at home.

2

Lower Your Blood Pressure with "Control Foods" and Nutritional Therapy

Your doctor has confirmed that your blood pressure is too high for your health. You are given prescribed medications. These are usually "water pills" or diuretics that help to wash out sodium from your body. Other nutrients may also be unwisely eliminated, and this could cause deficiency symptoms. A problem is that drug taking may become a permanent way of life. It may often interfere with body and, perhaps more seriously, with everyday foods. It becomes a dangerous "tug of war" in the battle to help lower your blood pressure.

A Nutritional Approach

To help correct your erratic or runaway blood pressure, your goal is to get to the cause: a metabolic error in your body. With the use of corrective nutrition along with "control foods," you can help keep your pressure in healthy check.

A Doctor's Eight-Step Program for Drugless Treatment of Mild Hypertension[1]

This approach has a double benefit: it lowers the blood pressure and it helps to control other risk factors for coronary heart disease, such as high blood cholesterol levels, adult-onset diabetes, and obesity. It could also save the person with slightly elevated blood pressure from a lifetime dependence on antihypertensive drugs, which often have troublesome side effects.

[1]Norman Kaplan, M.D., press release, May 2, 1985

15

This is the finding of Norman Kaplan, M.D., professor of internal medicine and chief of the hypertension unit at the University of Texas Health Science Center at Dallas. "I believe a non-drug approach should be the first treatment of mild hypertension, where the diastolic blood pressure is between 90 and 100 mm. Hg."

Dr. Kaplan bases his belief on the results of research done at the University and on a review of more than 160 published studies of the effects of weight loss, diet, mineral metabolism, exercise, and relaxation techniques.

Drugs: Proceed with Caution...Know the Risks Ahead

Dr. Kaplan explains, "The steadily growing tendency to treat even mildly hypertensive patients with drugs is bringing millions of non-symptomic people into lifetime drug therapy. For some, the risks of the drugs, as we have used them, may outweigh the benefits that can be gained from lowering the blood pressure," he warns.

"It is true that anti-hypertensive drugs will control the blood pressure. And that they have been shown to lower the death rate from stroke and heart failure that sometimes result from high blood pressure.

"But anti-hypertensive drugs have only spotty effects against what is by far the most serious and common complication of hypertension—coronary artery disease. I think we should consider all risk factors, along with the level of the blood pressure, before making the decision to use drugs."

The Doctor's Program You Can Follow at Home

Dr. Kaplan offers this eight-step drugless "prescription" for treating mild hypertension that he has found can work effectively for many people:

1. *Weight loss.* For the overweight, reduction should be the primary goal. The frequency of hypertension is about twice as high in the obese as in the nonobese; furthermore, even a small weight loss will often lower the blood pressure. The dual benefits of lowering blood

pressure and losing weight should provide incentive to stay on a weight-loss program.

2. *Sodium restriction.* For all hypertensive persons, salt in the diet should be restricted to 2 grams a day (about ½ teaspoon). This can be accomplished simply by leaving out salt in cooking and avoiding heavily salted foods such as smoked meats, pickles, and most canned and processed foods. After a few months on a lower-sodium diet, the taste preference for salty foods will decrease. However, to maintain calcium intake, the consumption of low-fat, low-sodium milk and cheese products should be continued.

3. *Fiber/fat in diet.* More high-fiber foods and less saturated fat in the diet are recommended for cholesterol-lowering diets. They may also help to lower your blood pressure.

4. *Alcohol.* In moderate amounts (less than 2 ounces a day) alcohol appears to protect against coronary heart disease. In larger amounts, it may raise the blood pressure enough to make it the most prevalent cause of reversible hypertension. Studies suggest that alcohol is responsible for at least 10 percent of hypertension in men and 1 percent of hypertension in women. A reasonable position would be to allow up to, but no more than, 2 ounces a day.

5. *Exercise.* After isotonic exercise such as walking, jogging, bicycling, or swimming, blood pressure falls as much as 25 percent and remains lower for at least 30 minutes. However, blood pressure may rise alarmingly during isometric exercise such as weight lifting. Regular active exercises of the isotonic type should be encouraged.

6. *Potassium.* For mild hypertension, potassium supplements are usually unnecessary. Potassium intake tends to increase when sodium is reduced, particularly by the substitution of natural foods for canned or processed foods.

7. *Other minerals.* Magnesium and calcium supplements should be given only to those who are deficient in the minerals until there is more evidence that they produce the desired results.

8. *Relaxation therapy.* Unfortunately, only a few hypertensives will choose to try relaxation therapy, and even fewer will stick with it. Most of those who do will achieve some lowering of blood pressure. A few will show a considerable decrease. In addition, they may be less anxious and feel better.

An Effective Pressure-Lowering Program

Dr. Kaplan notes, "This drugless therapy may lower the blood pressure to a level below 140/90 for a significant percentage of the large population with mild hypertension. Yet some patients may prefer treatment with drugs because it is easier and less expensive.

"Initial visits to a medical nutritionists and, for those older than 40, an exercise stress test before beginning a strenuous exercise program could make the expense of non-drug therapy slightly higher than medication.

"While the overall expense may be higher," says Dr. Kaplan, "the potential for improvement in overall health makes the cost seem trivial. Whether hypertensive patients take drugs to lower their blood pressure or not, they still need to lose weight, exercise regularly, eat a prudent diet and learn to relax. Non-drug therapies have a place in the treatment of all hypertensive patients."

LOWERS "DANGEROUS" BLOOD PRESSURE IN ELEVEN DAYS
ON DRUGLESS PROGRAM

Oscar B. was examined by his company physician and told the startling news that his blood pressure reading was a dangerously high 160/95. He was put on diuretics without delay but was sensitive to side effects such as an increase of uric acid in the bloodstream and also upset in blood sugar that could predispose him to diabetes.

Oscar B. wanted quick but safe treatment. He sought the help of a local nutrition-minded cardiologist who put him on the preceding eight-step drugless "prescription." Within four days, his pressure began to drop. By the end of the month, it had reached the safe reading of 120/80. Without drugs. Without the risk of side effects that could make the "cure" worse than the condition. It was with the use of this nutritional therapy program that helped to correct the metabolic disorder so that the body could become self-cured of this malfunction. He had been saved from this sneaky illness, thanks to nutritional therapy.

"Silent Executioner": The Misunderstood Illness

Hypertension is a condition without symptoms, a "silent executioner." It threatens the life and health of more persons than cancer. It is the nation's number two killer after heart disease. And one-half of those who have this disease are unaware of it.

18

The Numbers Game! Are You One of Them?

At least 40 million Americans have hypertension and over 20 million do not know it. It is aptly labeled a "silent executioner" because it does not make you feel sick. You may have it for years while it worsens until it strikes you down, often, in the prime of life!

No Relation to Tension

The name is somewhat of a misnomer. Hypertension is not nervous tension or anxiety. A very calm person may have the condition. The word is simply a medical term for high blood pressure.

What Is High Blood Pressure?

Blood pressure is the force of blood against the walls of the arteries and veins created by the heart as it pumps blood to every part of your body. When arterioles (small arteries that regulate blood pressure) contract, blood cannot easily pass through them. When this happens, your heart must pump harder to push the blood through. This increased push increases the blood pressure in your arteries. If the blood pressure increases above normal and remains elevated, the result is high blood pressure (hypertension).

How High Is Too High? As stated earlier, the danger is that you may have high blood pressure for years and never know it, because usually there are no symptoms. But pressure can be measured with a quick, painless test. The doctor uses a sphygmomanometer, a rubber cuff that is placed around your arm and then inflated with air. The cuff squeezes against and compresses a large artery in your arm, momentarily stopping the flow of blood.

As the air is released in the cuff and the blood begins to flow, the doctor listens with a stethoscope to the sound of the blood pushing through the artery. While listening and watching a gauge, the doctor records two measurements: (1) the pressure of blood flows when the heartbeats (systolic pressure) and (2) the pressure of the flow of blood between heartbeats (diastolic pressure).

Both numbers are then recorded as the blood pressure measurements, 120/80, for example, being considered a good reading: the first number listed is the systolic pressure (heart beating); the second number is the diastolic pressure (between beats). *Danger:* The more difficult it is for the blood to flow, the higher the numbers. You have hypertension if either number is consistently too high. *Example:* If the systolic pressure is over 160, it is considered elevated. If the diastolic pressure is above 90, you may be diagnosed as having high blood pressure.

Checklist of Danger Zones

Because both numbers go up and down together, most doctors and patients find it simpler to talk about just the diastolic reading. Here is a checklist of numbers designated as either "too high" ranging to "normal."

115 or above: you have severe hypertension, highly dangerous.

105–114: moderate hypertension.

95–104: mild hypertension.

90–94: borderline hypertension afflicting three out of every four people with high blood pressure.

80–89: a safe and normal zone, but new warning flags about a diastolic in the 80s could be a signal to start doing something now to prevent any increases.

Why Does It Happen?

It happens when there is too much pressure in your circulatory system. Your body has about 60,000 miles of blood vessels. Each time your heart beats (about 70 to 90 times each minute), blood is pushed through arteries, capillaries, and veins. The pressure of your heart's pumping action creates force on the walls of these vessels. Normal pressure pushes blood through the blood vessels. *Problem:* When arterial muscles tighten throughout the body and stay that way, or when "corrosion" such as cholesterol deposits accumulates on the inside walls, the result is high blood pressure.

What's the Blame?

It is found to be one's life-style. Possible causes include overweight. The more you weigh, the more cells your circulatory system must feed. This means it must work harder, under greater pressure, causing a rising in the numbers game.

Another cause is excess fat in the diet that leaves a coating of cholesterol on the blood vessel walls, which narrows the pathways through which the blood travels. As the coating builds up, it raises blood pressure and the risk of heart trouble.

Is Stress to Blame?

While seemingly calm people can have high readings, it is noted that unrelieved stress can be a culprit in elevated pressure. In reaction to daily stress, your mind sends your body into high gear. The higher your pressure at the onset, the higher the gear you go into and the greater the strain on your system. *Danger:* Untreated, this can cause a weakening of your arteries and lead to "brain overload" or stroke. Your heart or kidneys may rebel against working under this excessive pressure and fail! So we see that unrelieved or consistent stress could be a life-threatening risk.

The Risks You Face

When blood pressure is too great, blood vessels burst. If it happens in the heart, you may have a heart attack. If it's in the brain, you have a stroke. Blood on the brain has the same effect of turning a water hose on a pile of sand—the surface is rearranged and damaged. Continued pressure may also cause progressive damage to the kidneys. As arteries thicken and narrow, the amount of fluid the kidney can filter out is reduced. Some of the waste the kidney ordinarily would filter out into the urine will accumulate, eventually causing kidney failure.

We see that hypertension is the root cause of many premature deaths. But we are not without hope. The severity and fatality rate from all these hypertension-related afflictions may be lessened and, it is hoped, reversed and eliminated, with correction of molecular-biological errors of daily living. You *can* turn back the tide of mounting pressure and become a winner in the numbers game. Here is a set of nutritional therapies that could very well be a lifesaver in terms of bringing your pressure readings under control and into the safe zone.

The Magic Mineral That Controls
Blood Pressure

The evidence is small but dramatic—and growing. There is a link between blood pressure and the amount of calcium in your system. In various studies, it was found that if the diet contains adequate or abundant amounts of calcium, pressure readings are in the safe zone, even if the people are genetically disposed to the condition or are not salt watching. This "magic mineral" may well be a "natural medicine" to control your pressure readings.

How Calcium Keeps Pressure in Check

Calcium helps to modulate pressure by stabilizing the arterial blood flow. It exerts a bimodal benefit by balancing the rise in parathyroid hormone to regulate vascular smooth muscle tone and consequent blood pressure. Calcium has interactive aspects of metabolism with other nutrients. These responses tend to regulate blood pressure.

Salt-Washing Benefit

Calcium, together with potassium and other minerals, helps your body to slough off excess sodium or salt and protects you against an overload that could be a "nervous" trigger finger threatening to explode at any moment. Calcium also helps to wash salt out of your system. Calcium may be considered a "natural diuretic."

Calcium Balance = Pressure Balance

Calcium balance is the net of processes through which calcium enters and leaves your body. If you take in and absorb more calcium than you lose (through wastes), you are in *positive* calcium balance. If, on the other hand, you lose more than you take in, you are in *negative* calcium balance. *Danger:* if you remain in negative calcium balance for very long, your metabolism may accumulate sodium and deprive your circulatory system of the ability to maintain a safe and healthy arterial blood flow.

Nutritional Therapy:

Aim for a daily intake of adequate calcium from foods and/or supplements of 1,000 to 1,400 milligrams a day. (The recommended daily allowance or RDA of calcium for adults is 800. It is generally agreed that for safety's sake, boost intake to the 1,000–1,400 daily range.) Chart 2-1 presents some food sources of calcium.

You will do well, pressurewise, to plan your daily menu to include a variety of these foods to give you the needed calcium that will help to protect against an increase in life-threatening numbers.

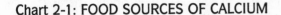

Chart 2-1: FOOD SOURCES OF CALCIUM

Food	Serving Size	Milligrams of Calcium
Skim milk	8 ounces	302
Low-fat (2%) milk	8 ounces	297
Whole milk	8 ounces	219
Buttermilk	8 ounces	285
Low-fat yogurt	1 cup	415
Low-fat yogurt with fruit	1 cup	314
Frozen yogurt	1 cup	200
Cottage cheese, creamed	1/2 cup	116
Swiss cheese	1 ounce	272
Parmesan, grated	1 ounce	390
Cheddar	1 ounce	204
Mozzarella	1 ounce	183
American cheese	1 ounce	174
Sardines with bones	3 ounces	372
Salmon with bones	3 ounces	285
Bean curd	4 ounces	154
Collards	1 cup	357
Turnip greens	1 cup	267
Kale	1 cup	206
Mustard greens	1 cup	193
Dandelion greens	1 cup	147
Broccoli	1 cup	136

CALCIUM THERAPY LIGHTENS PRESSURE, LENGTHENS LIFE SPAN

When told that her pressure was not only "moderately high" but "continuously climbing," Janet L. agreed to take chemical diuretics to wash out salt accumulation. This offered partial help but gave her side effects such as dizziness, irregularity, and nervous tremors. She sought the help of an endocrinologist who said that she could be able to lighten her pressure with the use of calcium. Janet L. gradually reduced diuretic use as she started to increase her calcium consumption. By aiming for 1,000 milligrams a day, she created the metabolic reaction that helped control her pressure. Within 16 days, she not only brought her pressure into the "safe zone" but was told her electrocardiogram showed she had the reading of a "young heart" at her age of 56 years! It was calcium that acted as a nutritional therapy to give her the blood pressure of a youth.

The Salt-Free Way To A Lower
Blood Pressure

Keep salt consumption under control, and you may well help develop immunity to high blood pressure.

The Salt Connection

There is a saying, "Water goes where the salt is." Because sodium clings to water, when an excessive amount enters the cellular fluid, it carries extra liquid with it. This extra liquid increases the volume of the plasma. To distribute the expanded blood, the heart must create additional pressure. It is forced to pump harder. This can elevate your pressure.

Taking a diuretic that pulls sodium and fluids from the tissues is one means of therapy. Anyone who has been on diuretics will complain of various side effects, of having sleep frequently disturbed by an emergency call from the bladder. This causes stress and a risk of pressure rise. To protect against this vicious cycle, it makes better sense to cut down or eliminate salt. This is a simple but effective nutritional therapy for high blood pressure.

How to Get Off the Salt Tightrope and
Lower Your Pressure

You'll discover new tastes formerly masked by salt. Your taste buds will sense the delicate variations of flavor in infinite and exciting varieties that have been lying undetected in your food, smothered by salt that formerly dominated the delicate character of food.

How Much Is Too Much?

The RDA for sodium is 1,100 to 3,300 milligrams (1/2 to 1-1/2 teaspoons) for adults. One teaspoon of table salt (5 grams) contains 2,200 milligrams of sodium. Therefore, your goal is to consume no more than about 1-1/2 teaspoons each day. Better yet, you will be doing your pressure a nutritionally therapeutic favor by adding *no* salt to your foods, before, during, or after cooking!

How to Shake the Salt Habit

- Add fresh grated lemon peel and herbs to plain yogurt as a dip for crisp raw vegetables.
- Blend lemon and/or orange juice with Neufchatel cream cheese and chopped ginger or unsalted nuts for an appetizer.
- Add citrus fruit juice and float thin lemon slices in vegetable-based soups and in beef, chicken, or tomato bouillon (no salt added).
- Add grated citrus peel and chopped parsley or chives to yogurt for garnish on broths or soups.
- Peel and slice or section fresh oranges or grapefruit for a fresh lettuce–onion salad.
- For oil and vinegar dressings, substitute 1/2 lemon juice and 1/2 herb-flavored vinegar for regular vinegar.
- Add thinly sliced unpeeled lemon to marinated cucumber salad.
- Blend orange-lemon juice with honey for fruit-cabbage combination.
- Blend lemon juice, dry mustard, and freshly ground black pepper. Serve as a spicy hot sauce for roasts, steaks, or chops.
- For marinades, blend lemon juice with herbs and honey.
- Add citrus juice to a barbecue sauce made of salt-free tomato paste, chili powder, honey, garlic, and onion.
- For baking or broiling, brush with a blend of oil, lemon juice, and poultry seasoning (salt-free); then dust with paprika.
- For baking whole fish, sprinkle inside and out with fresh lemon juice; then baste with lemon juice, chopped parsley, and unsalted butter or margarine.
- Dust fish pieces with flour mixed with grated lemon peel and herb mixture of sesame seed, oregano, basil, and thyme.
- For broiling fish, brush with melted salt-free butter or margarine, lemon juice, dill weed, or tarragon.

- Eating out? For a main dish, choose broiled, grilled, or roasted meat, fish, or poultry. Try to avoid those prepared or served with a sauce or gravy. Ask for a wedge or two of lemon for seasoning meat. Order plain steamed brown rice or a baked potato. Ask for salt-free butter or margarine, which many restaurants have on hand.

- When eating vegetables away from home, leave the juice in the bottom of the dish and eat only the solid pieces of vegetable to keep the salt to a minimum. *Tip:* A squeeze of juice from a lemon wedge also brings out flavor in most vegetables, including potato.

- At lunch time, roasted, broiled, or grilled meat, chicken, or turkey sandwiches will have minimum amounts of salt. *Avoid* pickles, olives, potato chips, and ketchup or other salty sauces.

- If you want a salad, ask for the chef's salad to be made with turkey or chicken meat only (omit highly-salted ham or cheese) and mix your own oil and vinegar or lemon juice dressing. If ordering the Diet Plate, ask for some fruit in place of the cottage cheese frequently provided. Avoid salted crackers or wafers.

- In someone's home, avoid the salted snack foods. If possible, tell the hostess you prefer not to have cured or salted meats or salted vegetables, but can have baked or broiled foods.

- Always, always read labels of packaged or prepared products. Many list sodium content. In many outlets, low-salt or salt-free products are available. If you must use such products, begin by reading labels and selecting salt-free items.

Throw Away the Salt—But Save the Shaker

Visit your local health store, herb and spice shop, or the spice rack at your market. Stock up on a variety of flavorful herbs and spices. Again, read labels, and avoid any product that contains salt. Get the smallest containers. Keep them in a cool, dry place. Use your shaker for garlic or onion powder (not salt!) which can be just as tasty as salt.

Salt-DANGER

Think of salt *not* as a flavoring but as sodium, a dangerous and potential detriment to your blood pressure and general health.

Chart 2-2 lists the average sodium content in a number of everyday foods. Plan ahead. Your blood pressure will be all the more grateful for it.

Chart 2-2: SODIUM CONTENT OF EVERYDAY FOODS

	Serving Size	Milligrams of Sodium
Beverages and Fruit Juices		
Cola, regular	1 cup	16
low calorie	1 cup	21
Coffee or tea	1 cup	1–2
Apple juice	1 cup	5
Orange juice, frozen	1 cup	5
Tomato juice	1 cup	878
Dairy Products		
American pasteurized processed cheese	1 ounce	406
Cheddar cheese	1 ounce	176
Cottage cheese, reg. and lowfat	1/2 cup	457
Swiss cheese	1 ounce	74
Milk, reg. and lowfat	1 cup	122
Pudding, instant chocolate	1/2	445
Yogurt, fruit flavored	1 cup	133
Eggs, Fish, Meat, Poultry, and Prepared Main Dishes		
Whole eggs	1 large	59
Black sea bass, raw	3 ounces	57
Mackerel, raw	3 ounces	40
Lake trout, raw	3 ounces	67
Tuna, light meat chunk canned in oil	3 ounces	303
white meat, low sodium	3 ounces	34
Shrimp, raw	3 ounces	137
canned	3 ounces	1,955
Beef, cooked, lean	3 ounces	55
Lamb, cooked, lean	3 ounces	58
Pork, cooked lean	3 ounces	59
bacon, cooked	2 slices	274
ham	3 ounces	1,114
Chicken, roasted drumstick with skin	1 drumstick	47
breast with skin	1/2 breast	69
Bologna, beef and pork	1 slice	224
Frankfurter	1 frankfurter	639
Chili con carne with beans canned	1 cup	1,194
Beef frozen dinner	1 dinner	998
Pizza with cheese	1/7 of 10" pie	367

Chart 2-2: (continued)

	Serving Size	Milligrams of Sodium
Fast Foods		
Cheeseburger	1	709
Shake	1	266
Fruit		
Apple	1 medium	2
Banana	1 medium	2
Orange	1 medium	1
Cantaloupe	1/2 melon	24
Peach	1 medium	1
Pineapple	1 cup	1
Watermelon, diced	1 cup	2
Grain Products, Breads, and Cereals		
White bread	1 slice	114
Whole wheat bread	1 slice	132
Cream of wheat cereal, reg.	1/4 cup	1
Mix'n eat	3/4 cup	350
Oatmeal, reg. or quick	3/4 cup	1
instant with maple and brown sugar	3/4 cup	277
Raisin Bran	1/2 cup	209
Corn Flakes	1 cup	256
Puffed Wheat	2 cups	2
Rice, regular white	1/2 cup	3
quick	1/2 cup	7
Rice, brown	1/2 cup	5
Stuffing mix	1 cup	1,131
Legumes and Nuts		
Baked beans, canned	1 cup	928
Dry, cooked navy beans	1 cup	3
Peanuts, dry roasted, salted	1 cup	986
unsalted	1 cup	8
Peanut butter, smooth or crunchy	1 Tbsp	81
Pecans	1 cup	1
Walnuts	1 cup	3
Soups		
Beef broth, cubed	1 cup	1,152
Chicken noodle condensed with water	1 cup	1,107
Mushroom, condensed with water	1 cup	1,031
Tomato condensed with water	1 cup	872
dehydrated with water	1 cup	943

Chart 2-2: (continued)

	Serving Size	Milligrams of Sodium
Vegetable condensed with		
water	1 cup	823
dehydrated with water	1 cup	1,000
Vegetables		
Beans, snap, cooked	1 cup	5
frozen	3 ounces	3
canned	1 cup	326
Broccoli, raw	1 stalk	23
frozen plain	3.3 ounces	35
Carrots	1 carrot	34
Corn cooked	1 ear	1
Frozen	1 cup	7
canned, cream style	1 cup	671
Lettuce	1 cup	4
Potatoes, baked or boiled	1 medium	5
Spinach cooked	1 cup	94
Squash, summer, cooked	1 cup	5
winter, frozen	1 cup	4
Tomato, raw	1 tomato	14
stewed	1 cup	584
Peas, frozen	3 ounces	80
Condiments, Fats, and Oils		
Baking powder	1 tsp	339
Baking soda	1 tsp	821
Catsup	1 Tbsp	156
Garlic powder	1 tsp	1
Garlic salt	1 tsp	1,850
Meat tenderizer	1 tsp	1,750
Monosodium glutamate (MSG)	1 tsp	492
Olives, green	4 olives	323
Pickles, dill	1 pickle	928
sweet	1 pickle	128
Barbecue sauce	1 Tbsp	130
Soy sauce	1 Tbsp	1,029
Worcestershire sauce	1 Tbsp	206
Vinegar	1/2 cup	1
Butter, regular	1 Tbsp	116
unsalted	1 Tbsp	2
Margarine, regular	1 Tbsp	140
unsalted	1 Tbsp	1
Oil, vegetable	1 Tbsp	0
Salad dressings		
blue cheese	1 Tbsp	153
French, bottled	1 Tbsp	214
Italian, bottled	1 Tbsp	116
Mayonnaise	1 Tbsp	78

Source: USDA Home & Garden Bulletin #233.

How Potassium Tames Your Runaway Blood Pressure

While you need to restrict sodium to soothe your blood pressure, these same "no-no" foods have potassium. This mineral is needed to maintain a normal flow of nerve signals and muscular contractions. Potassium plays an important role in energy release from carbohydrates, proteins, and fats. *Caution:* If you are taking diuretics or water pills, not only is sodium washed out but potassium is also eliminated. A deficiency could cause erratic heartbeats as well as disturbed blood pressure.

Nutritional Therapy

Plan for about 3,500 milligrams of potassium daily to help tame your runaway blood pressure. This magic mineral will enable your heart to pump blood with adequate force. Potassium will also strengthen the cellular walls and membranes to permit easier transportation of fluid and guard against water overload or edema. Keep your blood pressure in check with adequate daily intake of potassium-containing foods! This mineral may well be an all-natural "medicine" to protect against hypertension.

STABILIZES "THREATENING" PRESSURE IN SIX DAYS WITH POTASSIUM FOODS

When Martin J. was told he had a dangerously high pressure reading of 170/105, he followed a nutritional program as outlined by his doctor of osteopathy. But he still showed a too high reading. Further tests showed he had a serious potassium deficiency. To meet the "threat" of the "exploding" high pressure, he was told to boost intake of high-potassium foods. This simple nutritional therapy brought his pressure down to 130/90 within three days. By the end of the sixth day, his osteopathic physician happily told him the "wild" pressure was controlled and now he was at a more healthful 125/85. This *pressure-lowering mineral* snatched him from certain "jaws of death" with spiralling hypertension.

Had Your Potassium Today?

Chart 2-3 lists a variety of tasty everyday foods that are prime sources of this pressure-lowering mineral. Plan them as part of your daily menu, and you may well be master of your blood pressure, not the other way around.

Chart 2-3: POTASSIUM CONTENT OF EVERYDAY FOODS

Most of the items listed are good sources of potassium. A few such as fats, oils, processed cheese, eggs, and pizza are listed to show types of foods that tend to be low in potassium. The breads and rice are listed to show the difference between whole grain products. Note that a few items contain added salt and therefore are not recommended for sodium-restricted diets.

	Serving Size	Milligrams of Potassium
Beverages and Fruit Juices		
Grapefruit juice, frozen	1 cup	420
Orange juice, frozen	1 cup	503
Tangerine juice, frozen	1 cup	432
Tomato juice, low sodium	1 cup	549
Prune juice	1 cup	602
Dairy Products		
American pasteurized processed cheese*	1 ounce	23
Milk, whole	1 cup	351
skim	1 cup	355
Eggs, Fish, Meat, and Poultry		
Egg, whole	1 large	65
Tuna, chunk style, in water	3 ounces	237

	Serving Size	Milligrams of Potassium
Chicken, lt. meat without skin	3 ounces	369
Ground beef, lean, cooked	3 ounces	221
Pork loin, lean, cooked	3 ounces	280
Sirloin steak, lean, cooked	3 ounces	307
Fast Foods		
Pizza, frozen, cheese*	1/7 of 10" pie	65
Fruits		
Apricots, fresh, dried	3	301
	10 medium halves	343
Avocado	1/2	680
Banana	1 medium	440
Cantaloupe	1/2 melon	682
Dates, with pits	10	518

31

Chart 2-3: (continued)

	Serving Size	Milligrams of Potassium
Prunes	10 medium	448
Raisins, dark, not packed	2 Tbsp	138
Watermelon, diced	1 cup	160
Grain Products		
Bread, white*	1 slice	29
whole wheat*	1 slice	68
Oatmeal, cooked	1 cup	146
Rice, brown, cooked	1/2 cup	69
Rice, white, cooked	1/2 cup	29
Spaghetti, cooked	1 cup	103
Wheat germ	1 Tbsp	57
Legumes and Vegetables		
Broccoli, cooked	1/2 cup	207
Brussels sprouts, cooked	1/2 cup	212
Cauliflower, cooked	1/2 cup	129
Lentils, cooked	1/2 cup	249
Mushrooms, raw	1/2 cup	145

	Serving Size	Milligrams of Potassium
Peanuts, roasted with skins jumbo in shell	10	127
Potato boiled in skin	1 medium	556
Spinach, cooked	1/2 cup	292
Sweet potato, baked	1 large	342
Winter squash, baked	1/2 cup	473
Fats, Oils, and Sweets		
Butter*	1 Tbsp	3
Margarine*	1 Tbsp	3
Molasses, light	1 Tbsp	183
Oil	1 Tbsp	0

*These products contain significant amounts of added salt—see sodium listing.

Source: USDA Handbook #456.

How Onions and Garlic Create
Freedom from High Blood Pressure

Two tangy vegetables have long been used as folk remedies to help keep blood pressure in check. With the new knowledge of medical science as part of nutritional therapy, there is a sound basis for using these foods to protect against high blood pressure.

The Nutritional Therapy of Onions

A chemical analysis of onions will confirm the presence of prostaglandin Al, a hormonelike substance that definitely does lower blood pressure. This odoriferous root vegetable has oils that inhibit tumor growth in the laboratory. Onions also help to slow down platelet aggregation or clumping, which can lead to deadly blood clots or aneurysms traced to very high pressure.

The Nutritional Therapy of Garlic

This tangy vegetable is a concentrated source of allicin, a soothing ingredient. It is also rich in biologically active selenium, a mineral that prevents platelet adhesion and clot formation and thereby normalizes your blood pressure. Garlic has a dilating effect on the blood vessels, thereby causing a decided drop in the pressure. The aforementioned allicin is an active sulfur-containing compound that is changed into diallyldisulphide in the system to reduce the lipid (fat) levels in the serum (bloodstream) and liver and cause a biological chain reaction to bring down pressure.

Had Your Garlic and Onions Today?

Make it a daily program to include these two pressure-reducing vegetables in your nutritional plan. Since you will also be omitting salt, you will easily be able to substitute garlic and/or onions as a spicy substitute—and a pressure-saving combination, also!

Take charge of your blood pressure. Correct the nutritional errors with the use of these healthful foods and programs. You can make yourself immune to this "silent executioner" and avoid becoming one of the fatalities. Stabilize and keep stabilized your blood pressure readings with nutritional therapies.

IN REVIEW

1. A simple eight-step doctor-prescribed program, easily followed at home, can help to lower your blood pressure to a safe level, without any drugs or medications.

2. Oscar B. used this drugless "prescription" and normalized his "dangerous" pressure in 11 days.

3. Recognize the threat to your health that is caused by hypertension, the misunderstood illness that has no symptoms. No warning signs!

4. Go through the checklist of risk factors and make remedial adjustments.

5. Calcium is a "magic mineral" that helps to keep your pressure in check.

6. Using calcium foods, Janet L. lowered her pressure and lengthened her life span within 16 days.

7. Salt is a "no-no" on your pressure-lowering program. Follow the easy steps to getting off the salt tightrope and regulating pressure.

8. Potassium helps to tame your runaway blood pressure.

9. Martin J. stabilized "threatening" pressure in 6 days with tasty and lifesaving potassium foods.

10. Onions and garlic contain scientifically identified nutrients that expand blood vessels and control your pressure.

3

How to Feed Yourself a Forever Young Skin

Your skin is a reflection of your nutritional life-style. If you center your diet around fresh, wholesome foods, your skin is likely to radiate a youthful glow from within. If you upstage healthful foods with processed, chemicalized munchies, your skin loses its fresh appearance and looks as artificial and lifeless as the synthetics it is being fed. A forever young skin that is reasonably free of wrinkles, age spots, and sags is an inside job. By putting the proper foods and nutrients into your metabolism, you are able to nourish your skin so it glows healthfully. At any age!

Problem: Aging Wrinkles.
Solution: Nutritional Therapy

When skin becomes dry and loose, it shows creases that deepen into aging wrinkles. A lack or deficiency of oil production will dehydrate cells, and tissues beneath the surface of your body envelope to give your skin a parched appearance in the form of aging lines and wrinkles. To make up for deficiencies of important moisturizing sources, you need to use nutritional therapy from common everyday foods. You can then plump up and nourish your thirsty skin cells to give your face and body a youthful firmness, free of wrinkles.

Foods That Keep Your Skin in the Prime of Life

A number of everyday foods are brimming with nutrients that are able to perform a form of natural "face lifting" from within. Enjoy them daily and enjoy a skin that is kept in the prime of youthful life.

Vitamin A Will Erase Wrinkles

This nutrient helps protect against the clogging of pores that leads to blemishes and wrinkles. Vitamin A makes the cells lining the pores less

35

sticky. It makes the surface layer of the skin less "tough" or keratinizing and speeds up the life cycle of the cells, creating a continual sloughing effect to keep pores open.

Skin Rejuvenating Therapy. Vitamin A increases blood flow to the skin and stimulates skin cells (called fibroblasts) to make new connective tissue called collagen. This is the key to wrinkle prevention. Collagen is found in the supporting tissue just under the thin surface of the skin. A wrinkle is actually a crease in the collagen and skin. With vitamin A, the tiny creases and deep wrinkles may be erased, and your skin will take on a rejuvenating look.

Antiwrinkle Foods: Enjoy sweet potatoes, milk, carrots, winter squash, cantaloupes, liver, cheese, and eggs. These are prime sources of this valuable wrinkle-erasing vitamin A.

Nutritional Therapy: In a blender, combine 8 ounces milk, 4 ounces diced carrots, 2 teaspoons zucchini squash, 4 ounces cantaloupe. Whiz for 1 minute. Drink slowly to enjoy good taste. *Benefits:* the vitamin A will soon initiate the manufacture of collagen to plump up and firm your skin, to help protect against wrinkles.

Vitamin C for a Youthful Complexion

This nutrient is valuable for stimulating the growth of collagen, the cementlike substance that binds cells together to give you a firm skin. It also helps to strengthen elastin, the fiberlike substance synthesized by the body. It decreases and loses tone or elasticity as you age or when exposed to various stresses. It is vitamin C that helps to nourish the elastin and promote its continuous manufacture to help give you a youthful complexion even in later years.

Food Sources: Enjoy green peppers, kale, broccoli, oranges, grapefruits, strawberries, lemons, and limes.

Nutritional Therapy: Daily, have a fresh fruit salad with the important vitamin C foods. Also include the vegetables throughout the week. *Tip:* Break several vitamin C tablets (from health store) and sprinkle over your salad.

Vitamin E: Antiaging Therapy

The power of this vitamin is in its role as an antioxidant. It neutralizes harmful age-causing particles called free radicals and helps to wash them out of the system. Vitamin E has a biochemical ability to strengthen the tiny blood vessels in the lower layers of the skin. It constricts these capillaries, reduces their permeability, so less fluid leaks into surrounding tissues, and less aging occurs. This action also reduces surface skin temperatures by several degrees to create a slight, cooling effect. By helping to reduce the soft tissue damage by scavenging the free radicals, this vitamin helps to keep your skin (and body) younger and healthier.

Food Sources: Consider wheat germ oil, soybean oil, corn oil, safflower oil, and whole grain products such as whole wheat, bulgur, buckwheat, barley, oats, and wheat germ.

Nutritional Therapy: Switch to whole grain products and nonprocessed oils. *Tip:* Over a raw vegetable salad, sprinkle wheat germ and 2 tablespoons of oil. You will be giving your skin cells and capillaries a supercharging of vitamin E to cleanse away the age-causing free radicals and give you a youthful glow.

Zinc Zaps Age Signs

This lesser known mineral packs a powerhouse of rejuvenation for the skin by acting as a catalyst (helper) in many biological reactions. It boosts protein metabolism and makes the skin cells less likely to stick together, so there is a greater exchange of nutrients. It, too, performs as an antioxidant to devour and cast out the harmful age-causing free radicals. Zinc will help knock out and defuse aging signs from within your skin. It rebuilds collagen-elastin fibers to help give you that firm look of youth.

Food Sources: Consider wheat germ, wheat bran, cowpeas, skim milk, cheddar cheese, and nuts.

Nutritional Therapy: Blenderize 8 ounces of skim milk with 1 tablespoon wheat germ and 1 tablespoon wheat bran. Drink one glass each day to help put age-zapping zinc into your metabolism. *Tip:* Enjoy cooked cowpeas (blackeye) at least once a week with your regular salad or vegetable dish. Also have some nuts each day. A cheddar cheese sandwich several times a week is still another tasty way to give your metabolism the important zinc (and other vitamins and minerals) needed to rejuvenate your skin.

SIMPLE FOODS CREATE "NATURAL FACELIFT" IN NINE DAYS

When Grace O. heard herself being cruelly called "prune face" behind her back by snickering coworkers, she decided to do something about her deep furrows and wrinkles. She had tried everything, but the wrinkles just stared back at her in the mirror. She discussed plastic surgery with her dermatologist who suggested first trying nutritional therapy. She needed to correct the cause of her skin aging, namely, deficiencies of important cell-feeding nutrients.

Grace O. gave up processed foods and switched to wholesome, freshly prepared items. She boosted intake of the four wrinkle-erasing nutrients: vitamin A, vitamin C, vitamin E, and zinc. Within four days, her skin showed a more youthful color. At the end of two weeks, the crease lines and furrows became invisible. By the fourth week, this 56-year-old woman looked 20 years younger! Her coworkers wondered about her "secret," but she would keep it to herself. She had used nutrition to give herself a "natural facelift."

How to Drink Your Way to a Refreshingly Youthful Skin

Dry skin is a major cause of premature and unnecessary aging of the skin. You rarely find it on any chart of daily nutritional requirement, yet water is your body's most vital nutrient. Every cell in your body needs water to perform. Water helps to detoxify your body and skin of pollutants while providing essential moisture.

After the age of 35, skin becomes drier as the oil glands slow up activity. There is less oil-holding water in your cells. You need to protect yourself against this deficiency by drinking at least six to eight glasses of water each day.

Nutritional Therapy:

Increase intake of fresh fruits and vegetables (they range from 80 to 95 percent water), their juices, and herbal teas. In hot weather, drink an additional amount of water. You will be quenching the thirst of your cells, keeping them from dehydrating and giving you aged skin.

"No-No" Beverages

Be cautious about caffeine and alcohol. They are diuretics and cause you to lose water. Beverages high in sodium such as diet soft drinks or club soda (unless labeled caffeine and salt-free) can also raise your need for water because your body must maintain a constant balance of salt and water. *Best suggestion:* Ordinary water may well be your best moisturizing beverage.

HOW WATER THERAPY CORRECTED "GRANNY" SKIN

As a computer operator, Edna McG. was always kept busy. She may have neglected water intake, as her company physician suggested when she complained that while she was hardly in her fifties, her face and hands had "granny" skin. That is, wrinkled folds. She was advised to consume at least six glasses of water daily. "Make regular visits to the office water cooler" was the prescription! Edna McG. began this water program, stepped up with fresh fruits and vegetables. Within one month, the skin started to smooth out. Her face, throat, and hands, became youthful again. She could now pass for the thirties as a "young again" cover girl...thanks to water therapy!

How to Use Foods as Age-Reversing Skin Cosmetics

To give yourself the natural look, use wholesome foods as cosmetics and skin lotions. Here is a collection of nutritional therapies that work on the *outside* of your body to help reverse the aging process and give you the look and feel of youth.

Skin Toner

Clean your face well and rub with egg white. It will tighten on your skin and require plenty of rinsing, but it leaves your complexion rosy, glowing, immaculate, youthful.

Pore Cleanser

If you use powder or make-up base, be sure to remove it well before bedtime. Stale make-up clogs your pores and causes wrinkling and blemishes. Just use baby oil for removing makeup. It helps to moisturize your cells at the same time.

Enlarged Pores

Make a paste of oatmeal or cornmeal by mixing with a little water. Spread on your face and let remain for at least 15 minutes. Rinse with warm water and then cool water.

Oily Skin

Blend avocado to a paste and apply to your oily skin. Let remain 30 minutes and then splash off.

Wrinkled Eyelids

If too much work or television has your eyes feeling tired and your lids showing wrinkles, soak gauze in freshly squeezed orange juice and apply to your lids. Keep the gauze wet with juice and let remain on your lids about half an hour.

Crease-Age Lines...Anywhere

Cucumber turns up over and over as a nutritional therapy for skin. It is used as an ingredient in some expensive modern creams. Fashion models have this face-saving secret: rinse your face with cool water in which you have mashed some cut-up cucumber. It's refreshing and nutritious to the skin.

Dry Skin

Rub your face lightly with olive oil.

Wrinkles

The juice of a honeydew melon applied to wrinkles has been known to soften, moisturize, and smooth out the folds. Or mix mashed melon with petroleum jelly and spread on your face to fortify natural moisture.

Rough Hands

Wet oatmeal to paste consistency, rub over wrinkled parts of your hands (top or bottom), and let remain 20 minutes. Wash off.

Rough Elbows

Rest each elbow in half a grapefruit for a half hour.

Body Soak

Oil baths have been used by famous beauties for centuries—the ancient Greeks and Romans especially loved scented oils. Just pour 2 ounces of any oil in your bath water and luxuriate for a half hour. *Careful:* Avoid water that is too hot or too cold. Temperature extremes may shock your system and cause dryness too. Tepid water is best.

Fruit Facial

Rub a half lemon on your face and anywhere that you need firming up. It leaves your skin looking and feeling tingly clean and helps to remove excess oil.

Pep-Up Your Complexion

Lightly beat an egg white. Mix in 1 tablespoon of mayonnaise and 1 tablespoon of lemon juice. Spread over your face and throat and allow to dry. Rinse with warm water.

Wrinkle Eraser

Mix 1 egg white and ½ cup lemon juice with sufficient dry oatmeal to make a paste. Apply to face and neck and allow to dry. Rinse with warm water.

Dishpan Hands

Rub your hands with lemon juice after dishwashing to help restore the natural acid mantle of the skin which is removed in dishwater. (Without this natural acid condition, certain types of bacteria can grow and causes aging or dishpan hands.)

Dry, Scaly Skin

Lemon oils from the peel are perfect for helping to restore your skin to a silky soft feeling.

Face Scrub

Peel and mash a ripe avocado (one-half should be enough). Mix it with a half cup of yellow or white fine-grind cornmeal. Wash your face first, then apply the avocado-cornmeal paste onto the trouble spots. Gently rub in the mixture for a few minutes. Remove with a damp washcloth and splash off with witch hazel.

Night Cream

Work a piece of avocado (about the size of a strawberry) in the palm of your hand until it has a buttery consistency. Then take an equal amount of any night cream and mix the two together, blending well. Apply this vitamin-rich cream to your face and throat, massaging with your fingers. Let it remain overnight. Next morning, your skin will glow with vitality and freshness.

Watermelon Lotion

Cut a slice of chilled, ripe watermelon, force it through a sieve and catch the juice in a bowl. Strain and put the liquid in a jar. Pat on your face and neck. Let remain until dry, about 5 minutes; then splash off with cool water.

These nutritionally therapeutic creams and lotions will help reverse the aging tide and give your skin a second chance to recover and retain its second youth!

"Forever Young Skin Food Tonic"

Troubled with dark circles under your eyes? Worried about deepening lines and creases on your face, throat, and elsewhere? Skin starting to sag? Do you look and feel old before your time? The reason may be in a deficiency of a vitamin group that stands head and shoulders above all others in terms of keeping your skin young.

The B-Complex Vitamin Family

A deficiency of just one of these vitamins can give you blotchy, lifeless, or blemished skin. The B-complex vitamins are needed to protect against scaly conditions of the skin and nerve deterioration. These vitamins activate enzyme systems required for the complete metabolism of carbohydrate foods needed to energize your skin and body cells. The B-complex family will activate metabolic reactions involved in oxidation-reduction processes to help give you a youthful skin.

If your skin looks older than you want it to, you could be in need of these vitamins. You can give your entire metabolism a supercharging of energy to firm up your skin cells with a simple but powerfully effective Forever Young Skin Food Tonic. Just drink one glass a day. See the results almost from the start.

The "Tonic"

Combine 8 ounces of orange juice with 2 tablespoons brewer's yeast powder; add 1 teaspoon lecithin granules, 1 teaspoon wheat germ, 1 teaspoon vegetable oil. Blenderize for 2 minutes. Drink slowly *before* breakfast so nutrients can work without interference from other foods.

Skin-Saving Benefits:

The vitamin C from the orange juice activates the B-complex treasure from the brewer's yeast and lecithin to combine with the vitamin E from the wheat germ and vegetable oil. In combination, this tonic will nourish your membranes, strengthen the cartilage and connective tissue, preserve oxygen within your skin cells, improve collagen-elastin stability, and lubricate and regenerate your entire skin.

The rich concentration of B-complex vitamins in this Forever Young Skin Food Tonic makes it a powerhouse of nutritional therapy from within.

LOOKS 10–20–30 YEARS YOUNGER WITH TONIC

When Helen LaR. was mistaken as the older sister of the three at a high school reunion (she was the youngest by nine years!), she decided to do something about her prematurely aging skin. She sought the help of a nutritionist who was known for aiding others who had skin disorders. The nutritionist suggested a return to fresh, wholesome foods and the use of the Forever Young Skin Food Tonic. Each day, for three weeks, Helen LaR. followed this easy plan. Quickly, her sallow complexion became fresh and young looking. Wrinkled folds started to smooth out. Crease lines just went away. Even more astounding was her boosting of energy in body and mind. She not only looked younger, but she felt more vibrant and alive. By the end of the month, she had such a young looking skin that radiated freshness, she was again mistaken by a neighbor, but this time, she was thought to be a "daughter" of one of her sisters!

Problem: Unsightly Red Veins on Skin

Nutritional Therapy: Turn to bioflavonoids

In this condition, tiny red threadlike veins have laced themselves across the face, most often on the lower cheeks. The cause may be traced to capillary fragility which creates these small red veins, running like wheel spokes beneath the skin. This suggests a weakness in your blood-carrying veins. Because of the damaged walls, fluid leaks through into areas beyond the veins.

To correct the problem from a nutritional view, the bioflavonoids (vitamin C complex with rutin, another nutrient) are needed to help strengthen this entire area.

Dietary Improvement

Boost your intake of bioflavonoid-rich foods such as citrus fruits, rose hips, turnip greens, green peppers, cabbage, and buckwheat (a prime source of rutin). *Tip:* The stringlike netting found near the inner peel of grapefruits, oranges, and tangerines is a concentrated source of bioflavonoids. Eat the whole fruit, including these strings to give your capillaries a powerhouse of bioflavonoids and protect against as well as reverse your problem of unsightly red veins.

How Oils Can Rebuild Your Skin from Head to Toe

With the use of fish liver oils, you can give your entire body a youthful skin all over. Fish oils are prime sources of vitamins A and D and contain the essential fatty acids that exert a powerful influence within your metabolism to prime your youth pump. This can be seen if you are in your late thirties and are concerned about aging skin. Let us see how this works.

Why Your Skin Ages

Your dermis (the supporting tissue lying beneath the paper-thin top layer of skin) contains water, fat, and spindly, star-shaped cells called fibroblasts. These cells act to support your network fibers, collagen, and elastin, to give your skin firmness and elasticity. But starting in the thirties, your dermis absorbs less water and fat. Your skin loses its firm and plump appearance. Oil-producing cells start to slow down. Your skin gets drier. Cell renewal begins to slow down, particularly in the menopausal stage. New cells do not develop as quickly. The older ones remain longer on your skin surface. Fibroblast cells produce fewer supporting fibers. Whatever is produced has less resiliency than in young skin. Your body envelope receives less oxygen and fewer nutrients as small capillaries beneath the surface start to close off.

Nutritional Therapy

Aging alone is not the cause of skin changes. Rather, how fast and how strong such changes occur depend largely on your nutritional intake. If you are adequately nourished, you may be able to cope with changes with fewer age signs. With the use of specific nutrients, vitamins A and D and essential fatty acids, you may be able to meet the challenges—and win. You can do it with fish liver oils. They contain these valuable nutrients which are able to stimulate your fibroblasts to create more essential fibers to support your skin structure. These vitamins combine with the fatty acids to provide valuable moisture to guard against dryness. They further introduce important oxygen so that your small capillaries can remain open and function to admit the free passage of nutrients. With the use of fish liver oils, you may well help rebuild your skin from head to toe.

Take Two at Bedtime...Look Younger in the Morning

About 30 minutes before bedtime, take 2 tablespoons of fish liver oil with water, milk, or citrus juice. Feel yourself relax. Then turn in. Throughout the night, your metabolism will seize hold of the important fibroblast-strengthening nutrients and begin to rebuild and repair your skin. This is an inside job. By morning, you should start to look and feel younger. Sagging skin, bags under the eyes, wrinkles, and unsightly blemishes will gradually ease and soon become erased with this inner rebuilding process.

Fish liver oil may well be the most valuable skin-feeding nutritional therapy you will need to help give your skin a second start in life!

Put the Skin-Aging Process on Hold

You have seen the reactions when former classmates get together at a class reunion after 20 years. As you greet a long-absent friend and notice the lined face, the changes that have made her look "so old," you cannot help but ask yourself silently, "Do I look that old, too?" The answer is in an honest self-appraisal before the mirror. The next step is to decide to put your aging process on hold as you begin a program of nutritional therapy. You do *not* have to accept your face and body skin the way it is. You *do* have an alternative with the use of corrective nutrition, inside and outside. You *can* have a younger skin, at any age!

WRAP-UP

1. Vitamin A has antiwrinkling and skin-rejuvenating powers that work swiftly.

2. Use a vitamin C boost to give yourself a youthful complexion.

3. Halt skin aging with the use of vitamin E.

4. Zinc will zap age signs and rebuild collagen-elastin fibers, the key to a youthful skin.

5. Grace O. used everyday foods to give herself a "natural facelift" in a short time.

6. Water therapy corrected Edna McG.'s "granny" skin very quickly.

7. Simple foods can be used as cosmetics to cleanse pores, correct dry-oily skin, smooth wrinkled eyelids, erase crease-age lines, soften rough hands and elbows, and brighten complexion.

8. The Forever Young Skin Food Tonic is a powerhouse of nutrients that firm up your skin, almost immediately.

9. Helen LaR. took 10-20-30 years off her face with the tonic.

10. Fish liver oils are rich, concentrated sources of nutrients that guard against and reverse the aging process. Just 2 tablespoons at bedtime and you wake up looking and feeling younger in the morning.

4

Cancer: How to Use Nutritional Safeguards to Build Your Resistance

Can vitamins halt the growth of tumors or shrink existing ones? Can nutritional therapy be used to keep cancer patients alive longer? Can specific foods be used to build immunity to cancer?

Chemoprevention—the use of nutrition to resist the start of cancer—is making it possible to fight back against this threat and win the battle with the use of a group of potent nutrients in foods. By making some simple adjustments in your daily food program, you can reduce the risks of developing cancer. You also can help to turn around certain existing cancer growths, block its spread, and resist the threatening consequences.

A major breakthrough in the search for dietary correction of the cancer threat has been announced by the National Academy of Sciences in a major report.[1] Nutritional therapies call for eating less fat; very little of salt-cured, pickled, and smoked foods; and more fruits, vegetables, and whole grains. The panel of experts from the Academy further urged daily consumption of fruits and vegetables rich in beta-carotene, the predecessor of vitamin A as well as vitamin C, which was found to inhibit the formation of certain cancer-causing substances and also lower the risk of cancers of the stomach and esophagus. With this set of guidelines, it was noted in various tests, that nutrition would be able to protect against specific cancers. It could also help undo much damage if cancer already did take hold. Nutritional therapy could even heal or "cure" some cancer.

[1]*Diet, Nutrition and Cancer,* National Academy of Sciences, Washington, D.C., 1982.

47

Correct Nutrition Can Give You
Immunity to Cancer

Scientists have noted that:

1. Eighty percent of all cancers may be related to the environment, and to things you eat, drink, or smoke rather than to factors you cannot control such as family background. If you change the things you can control, there is strong evidence you can reduce your risk of getting cancer.

2. Thirty-five percent of all cancer deaths may be related to the way you eat. Make an adjustment in your dietary program, and you have build stronger resistance to cancer. You may even be able to knock out and defuse the cancer infestation and win the battle against this major killer.

Based on evidence at hand, you may win the battle by following a set of simple guidelines as issued by the American Cancer Society.

Seven-Step Nutritional Program to
Build Cancer Immunity

1. *Avoid obesity.* Sensible eating habits and regular exercise will help you avoid excessive weight gain. There is a higher cancer risk among overweights, particularly if you are 40 percent overweight. Your risk increases for colon, breast, and uterine cancers. Tests indicate that the incidence of cancer is reduced and the life span lengthened by maintaining an ideal weight. Are you obese? Shedding those excess pounds may be one way to lower cancer risk.

2. *Cut down on total fat intake.* Excess intake of fats increases the chances of developing certain cancers like the breast, colon, and prostate cancers. Americans consume about 40 percent of total calories as fat. A decrease in the amount of fat to 30 percent of total calories, on the average, will help protect against this threat. You will also be able to control your body weight more easily.

3. *Eat more high-fiber foods.* Fiber is a term used to cover food components not readily digested in the human intestinal tract. These substances, abundant in whole grains, fruits, and vegetables, consist largely of complex carbohydrates of diverse composition. It

is believed that bulky, undigested food residues make quicker passage through the intestines, thus reducing the time in which bacteria or other cancer-causing substances could be in contact with intestinal tissues. (Fiber is also defined as the residue of plant cells after digestion by alimentary enzymes.) If bile acids or their breakdown products might be involved in causing cancer, the high-fiber diet with its larger bulk would decrease the time such agents could be in contact with intestinal tissues. Fiber may change the composition of bacterial flora and its interaction with carcinogens.

4. *Include foods rich in vitamins A and C in your daily diet.* Dark green and deep yellow vegetables and fruits such as carrots, spinach, yams, peaches, apricots, tomatoes, and cantaloupes are rich in beta-carotene, a form of vitamin A, that may reduce the risk of cancers of the larynx, esophagus, and lung. Second, oranges, grapefruit, strawberries, green and red peppers, lemons and melons contain ascorbic acid or vitamin C, which inhibits the formation of nitrosamines in the stomach. (Nitrosamines are powerful carcinogens formed when nitrates found in pickled items, in cured and preserved meats, combine with protein.) These two nutrients appear to offer protection or modify the incidence of stomach and esophageal cancer.

5. *Include cruciferous vegetables in your daily meal plan.* Cruciferous vegetables belong to the mustard family, whose plants have flowers with four leaves in the pattern of a cross. Some epidemiologic studies suggest that daily consumption of these vegetables may reduce the risk of cancer, particularly of the gastrointestinal and respiratory tracts. These vegetables include cabbage, broccoli, Brussels sprouts, kohlrabi, cauliflower, rutabaga, and turnips. These same cruciferous vegetables are prime sources of fiber as well as other vitamins and minerals, making them all-around healthful foods.

6. *Eat moderate amounts of salt-cured, smoked, and nitrate-cured foods.* Conventionally smoked foods such as hams, some varieties of sausage, and fish absorb some of the tars that arise from incomplete combustion. These tars contain numerous carcinogens that are similar chemically to the carcinogenic tars in tobacco smoke. The risks may apply primarily to conventionally smoked meats and fish. These processed foods may increase the risk of cancer of the esophagus and stomach. There is evidence that nitrate and nitrite can enhance nitrosamine formation, both in foods and the digestive

tract. Nitrate is used for meat preservation to prevent botulism (food poisoning) and to provide color and flavor.

7. *Keep alcohol consumption moderate if you do drink.* The heavy use of alcohol, especially when accompanied by cigarette smoking or chewing tobacco, increases risk of cancers of the mouth, larynx, throat, esophagus, and stomach. Alcohol abuse can result in cirrhosis, which may lead to liver cancer.

With the American Cancer Society's seven-step guideline, you may well be able to use nutritional therapy to prevent cancer or reverse its spread and free yourself from becoming another statistic in the list of fatalities.

Cancer: What Is It? Who Gets It? Who Will Survive?

What Is It?

Cancer is a disease characterized by uncontrolled growth and spread of abnormal cells. If the spread is not controlled or checked, it can be fatal.

Who Gets It?

It strikes at any age. It kills more children 3 to 14 than any other disease. It strikes more frequently with advancing age. Over 450,000 will die yearly of cancer—1,266 people a day, about one every 68 seconds. About 71 million Americans now living will eventually have cancer. Over the years, cancer will strike in approximately three out of four families. In an average year, about 910,000 people will be diagnosed as having cancer.

Who Will Survive?

Over 5 million Americans today have a history of cancer, 3 million of them with diagnosis five or more years ago. Most of these 3 million can be considered cured, while others still have evidence of cancer. By "cured" is meant that a patient has no evidence of disease and has the same life expectancy as a person who never had cancer. Today, about 340,000 Americans, or 3 out of 8 patients who get cancer, will be alive five years after diagnosis.

(The decision as to when a patient may be considered cured is one that must be made by the physician after examining the individual patient. For most forms of cancer, five years without symptoms following treatment is the accepted time. However, some patients can be considered cured after one year, others after three years, whereas, some have to be followed much longer than five years.)

THE SEVEN-STEP NUTRITIONAL THERAPY PLAN TO PROTECT AGAINST COLON CANCER

When Andrew J. was told by his proctologist that since several family members had colon cancer, he was at high risk, he understandably became frightened. He had three youngsters in school, a newly purchased home, a supervisor's job with a future. Would he face the hereditary risk of being cut down in the prime of his life? Colon cancer caused about 60,000 deaths in a typical year, second only in incidence to that of lung cancer. What were his chances?

His proctologist eased his panic by explaining that the proctosigmoidoscopy exam showed he could build a form of immunity if nutritional therapy were begun. He gave Andrew J. the American Cancer Society's seven-step plan and suggested he add another step by eliminating smoking and also cutting down all drinking. Eager to avoid the risk, he followed the program. Four months later, a new exam showed his colonic area to be in the best of health. The seven-step nutritional therapy plan now became his permanent way of life. It also gave him permanent life, he would say happily.

How Nutrients Build Immunity to Risk of Cancer

To build resistance to the risk of cancer, consider nutritional therapy. Some nutrients appear to act as anticancer fighters to correct the malfunction responsible for molecular chaos. You may want to build immunity with emphasis on one or more of these individual groups. This form of nutrition may well turn the tide against the risk of the spread of cancer and build a form of natural immunity.

Vitamin A or Beta-carotene

A report issued by the Nutrition Support Service of the Hospital of the university of Pennsylvania offers hope for immunity with this nutrient.[2] Robert C. Fried, M.D., explained that beta-carotene is called a provitamin because, once ingested, it is converted to vitamin A by the body's

---

[2]Clinical Nutrition Newsletter, University of Pennsylvania, Philadelphia, August, 1984.

tissues. It acts as a cancer inhibitor in many situations. It nourishes the epithelial varieties of tissues (those involving the cellular covering); it helps to shrink tumors, especially in epithelial cancer; additionally, beta-carotene offers defensive immunity to protect against the recurrence of the same cancer.

Vitamin C

Dr. Fried also explained that the risk of developing certain cancers (particularly gastric and esophageal carcinogens) could be reduced with regular intake of this vitamin. It inhibits the formation of carcinogenic N-nitroso compounds that have been found to be the villain in gastrointestinal cancers. It also appears that indols (a protein product containing tryptophan) from vegetables stimulate the increased manufacture of aryl hydrocarbon hydroxylases, which act as barriers to various cell-damaging chemicals. The doctor feels that boosting intake of vitamin C from vegetable sources is one way by which you can fortify yourself with internal protection against cancer. Typical food sources include turnip greens, kale, broccoli, green peppers, Brussels sprouts, cauliflower, cabbage, and tomatoes.

Vitamin E

"With various nutrients, we have for the first time in human history a biological tool to prevent cancer," says Kedar N. Prasad, Ph.D., a researcher at the University of Colorado Health Sciences Center and president of the International Association for Vitamins and Nutritional Oncology. "And the prospects for treatment with nutrients look promising as well. It will take a long time before we have conclusive evidence of all the anti-cancer properties of these substances, but we've made a good start."

Investigators at the University of Colorado have discovered in laboratory tests that vitamin E may halt the growth of prostate cancer cells. Test tube research had already shown that vitamin E could kill or inhibit other kinds of malignant cells, but this study zeroes in on vitamin E's impact on cancer of the prostate.

"Our data suggest," says Dr. Prasad, "that vitamin E may be useful in the treatment of patients with prostate cancer. After all, compared to cancer drugs, vitamin E is very low in toxicity so it can be easily incorporated into chemotherapy treatments. It simply will not interfere with standard therapy."[3]

How Vitamin E Builds Immunity. By helping cell membranes remain healthy, this vitamin appears to guard genetic material from damage that could lead to cancerous changes. Vitamin E intercepts and neutralizes dangerous molecular fragments, called oxidants, that might otherwise penetrate the nuclei and alter the DNA of healthy cells. This could predispose one to dangerous forms of cancer. It is vitamin E that acts to build internal immunity against the risk of this molecular damage. It has been found that this vitamin helps to prevent chromosome damage in cells exposed to certain chemicals. It also appears to be beneficial in building resistance to a common breast disease called fibrocystic cancer, affecting about 50 percent of all women who have a two- to eightfold greater risk of developing breast cancer.

Selenium

This mineral is a potent antioxidant that protects the cell membrane from free-radical or oxidant attack. Dr. Richard A. Passwater hails this mineral in his book, *Selenium as Food and Medicine,* as a barrier against the risk of cancer.[4] Selenium helps to produce an enzyme called glutathione peroxidase, or GSH-Px, for short, notes Dr. Passwater. He explains that here is a valuable antioxidizing enzyme that protects your body from damage by free radicals—the substances that bombard and break down cells and may trigger cancer. Selenium comes to the rescue by entering your red blood cells. It stimulates your immune system. It further alters the workings of carcinogenic substances, protecting against an accumulation of dangerous free radicals. The current RDA for selenium is 50 to 200 micrograms a day. You may want to aim for about 150 micrograms as a protective supply of needed GSH-Px. You will find 102 micrograms in ½ cup of water-packed tunafish. (The same serving packed in oil gives you only 55 micrograms.) One slice of whole wheat bread has 18 micrograms. Other rich sources are liver, kidneys, Brazil nuts, and brown rice. *Caution:* because of the potential toxic risk of selenium overdose, the *medically*

---

[3]*Prevention* magazine, Emmaus, Pa., June 1985.
[4]*Selenium as Food and Medicine* by Dr. Richard A. Passwater, Keats Publishing Co., New Canaan, Conn., 1980.

unsupervised use of selenium as a food supplement cannot be recommended.

HOW MIRIAM F. USED NUTRITIONAL THERAPY

Miriam F. became understandably concerned when her gynecologist, who had learned of her family's history of breast nodules, told her she would have to build resistance to cancer without delay. Miriam F. discussed nutritional therapy with the surgeon who explained that tests showed she had low levels of both vitamin E as well as selenium. By boosting intake of foods containing these nutrients, Miriam F. could help build immunity to offset the risk of so-called heredity cancer.

She followed a simple program that called for an increased consumption of vitamin E foods from unrefined wheat germ oil, whole grain breads and cereals, nuts, and seeds. She also consumed more brown rice as well as about 2 cups of water-packed tunafish throughout the week. A few diced Brazil nuts mixed in a whole grain cereal would give her both these nutrients. Results? By the end of the month, these immunity-building nutrients helped to improve her resistance. A new exam showed Miriam F. to be in excellent health and not the slightest risk of growths.

Two Potential Immunity Builders

Both vitamin E and selenium help the workings of an intracellular messenger, cyclic AMP, to become broken down by an enzyme, phosphodiesterase, as soon as signals are sent into the cell. These nutrients protect against any blockage of the cyclic-AMP signal, thereby guarding against the runaway proliferation of tissues.

How To Plan Your Food Choices To Help Build Your Resistance Against Cancer

Here is a set of dietary guidelines that will help to prevent and treat certain types of cancer. Nutritional therapy is one part of your total health picture. Daily exercise, not smoking, maintaining ideal weight, keeping yourself safe on the job, and having regular physical checkups add up to total resistance to cancer and other illnesses.

Dietary Fiber

Choose more often whole grain products such as:

- Bakery products, including whole wheat crackers; bran muffins; brown, rye, oatmeal, pumpernickel, bran, and corn breads; whole wheat English muffins, bagels.
- Breakfast cereals such as bran cereals, shredded wheat, whole grain · or whole wheat flaked cereals, others that list dietary fiber content.
- Other foods made with whole grain flours such as waffles, pancakes, pasta, and taco shells.
- Foods made with whole grain such as barley, buckwheat groats, and bulgur wheat.
- Fruits such as apples, pears, apricots, bananas, berries, cantaloupes, grapefruit, oranges, pineapples, papayas, and prunes, raisins.
- Vegetables such as carrots, broccoli, potatoes, corn, cauliflower, Brussels sprouts, cabbage, celery, green beans, summer squash, green peas, parsnips, kale, spinach, other greens, yams, sweet potatoes, and turnips.
- All dry peas and beans such as black, kidney, garbanzo, pinto, navy, white, and lima beans.
- Lentils, split peas, and blackeyed peas.
- Snack foods include fruits and vegetables, unbuttered popcorn, whole grain and bran cereals, and whole grain breads and crackers.

Choose less often:

- Refined bakery and snack products such as refined flour breads, quick breads, biscuits, buns, croissants, snack crackers and chips, cookies, pastries, and pies.

Your Fat Program

Choose more often:

- Lower-fat poultry such as chicken, turkey, and Rock Cornish hens (without skin).
- Fresh or frozen fish or water-packed canned fish.
- Beef, veal, or lamb with little or no marbling (visible intermixed fat) and trimmed of all fat.
- Peas and beans such as pinto, black, kidney, garbanzo, navy, white, lima beans; lentils; and blackeye and split peas.

- Lower-fat dairy products such as skim milk and buttermilk, low-fat yogurt.
- Skimmed evaporated milk, nonfat dry milk.
- Low-fat cheese such as ricotta, pot, farmer, or cottage, and mozzarella, or cheeses made from skim milk.
- Sherbet, frozen low-fat yogurt, and ice milk.
- Low-fat salad dressings.
- Low-fat margarine.

Choose less often:

- Higher-fat poultry such as duck and goose, chicken with skin.
- Frozen fish sticks, tuna packed in oil.
- Fatty luncheon meats, bologna, hot dogs, and sausage.
- Beef, veal, and lamb cuts with marbling, untrimmed of fat.
- Peanut and other nut butters.
- Trail mix.
- Full-fat dairy products such as whole milk, butter, and yogurt made from whole milk.
- Sour cream, sweet cream, half and half, whipped cream, and other creamy toppings (including imitation).
- Full-fat soft cheeses such as cream cheese, cheese spreads, Camembert, and Brie.
- Hard cheeses such as cheddar, Swiss, bleu, American, Jack, and Parmesan.
- Ice cream.
- Coffee creamers, including nondairy.
- Cream sauces, cream soups.
- Shortening, lard, meat fats, salt pork, and bacon.
- Mayonnaise.
- Margarine.
- Gravies, butter sauces.
- Snacks such as donuts, pies, pastries, cakes, cookies, brownies, and croissants.

- Potato chips and snack crackers.
- Canned puddings, icings, candies made with butter, cream, and chocolate.
- Avoid food preparation methods such as batter and deep-fat frying or sauteeing. Avoid use of fatty gravies and sauces. Do not add cream or butter to vegetables.

Your Vitamin A and C Program

Choose any of the following:

- Dark green leafy vegetables such as broccoli, Swiss chard, kale, spinach, romaine, endive, chicory, escarole, watercress, collard, beets, turnips, and mustard and dandelion greens.
- Vegetables such as asparagus, green and red peppers, cauliflower, cabbage, Brussels sprouts, bean sprouts, mushrooms, squash, green beans, onions, okra, and tomatoes.
- Yellow-orange vegetables such as carrots, sweet potatoes, pumpkins, and winter squash.
- Yellow-orange fruits such as apricots, cantaloupes, similar melons, cherries, papayas, peaches, prunes (even though they are not yellow in all forms), berries, pineapples, plums, strawberries, and watermelons.
- Citrus fruits like lemons, limes, oranges, tangerines, and grapefruit.
- Juices made from any of the foregoing.

Your Vitamin E Program

Choose any of the following:

- Wheat germ oil, whole grain products, vegetable oils, sunflower seeds, raw or sprouted seeds, nuts and grains, and green leafy vegetables.

Your Selenium Program

Choose any of the following: tunafish, water-packed; fresh garlic; barley; whole wheat bread; egg noodles; brown rice; beef liver; beef kidneys; Brazil nuts.

Can Nutritional Therapy "Knock Out" Cancer?

Can nutritional therapy disarm dangerous cancers? The new knowledge of using nutrients as weapons does suggest you can help to build immunity to the risk of the formation of misshapen cells and the onset of cancer. These same nutrients are able to "knock out" enemy cells and mend injuries to help free you from cancer.

Your Hope for Health

The facts show that about 3 out of every 10 cancer deaths are traced to poor diet. Fortify your resistance with the use of the preceding seven-step program and you will enjoy better health and freedom from the risk of cancer.

SUMMARY

1. Since 8 out of all 10 cancers are environmentally related and 3 out of 10 cancers are diet connected, you can build immunity with proper self-care.
2. The easily followed seven-step nutritional program should be your foundation of better health.
3. Andrew J. was able to resist colon cancer with this improved program.
4. Boost intake of four nutrient groups to build an inner fortress against cancer.
5. Miriam F. used two nutrients in everyday foods to build immunity to the threat of heredity-caused breast cancer.
6. Plan your anticancer diet program with suggested guidelines.
7. You can be victorious in the threatening battle against cancer with nutritional therapy.

The Low-Fat Way to a Healthier and Younger Heart

When you hear the saying, "The way to a person's heart is through the stomach," do you immediately plan imaginary menus? Do you think of rib-eye steak, baked potato with cheese and bacon, vegetables with hollandaise sauce, and cheesecake? Or do you think of chicken-fried steak with cream gravy, fresh snap beans flavored with salty fat, and banana cream pie with whipped cream?

The condemned man's last meal! Either menu could lead to a man's heart—or his heart attack! Both are laden with cholesterol-rich foods and saturated fats that could trigger heart disease. It could very well be the man's last meal.

Cholesterol and Fat—Are You Eating Too Much?

All persons 2 years of age and older need to make nutritional adjustments to reduce the risk of heart trouble, according to a panel of experts at the National Institutes of Health (NIH). In particular, it is lifesaving to control intake of both cholesterol and fat.

Cholesterol-Control Goal

Lower your blood cholesterol to the NIH-recommended 180 milligrams or less for those age 30 and younger; 200 milligrams or less for those over age 30. Reduce your blood cholesterol by about 10 percent. Consume no more than 300 milligrams of dietary cholesterol each day.

Fat-Control Goal

Lower total fat levels by limiting fat intake to no more than 30 percent of total calories. Plan to consume one-third from animal sources and two-thirds from vegetable and plant sources. *Example:* on a 2100-calorie-a-day diet, as much as 630 calories may come from fats. (Because 1 gram of fat contains 9 calories, fat intake comes to 70 grams, or 2.5 ounces.)

How to Reach a Fat Balance. According to the NIH guidelines, no more than 10 percent of the total calories intake (about 210 calories) should come from saturated fats, found mostly in animal and dairy products. The rest, about 420 calories, should be shared between polyunsaturated fats, such as vegetable oils, and monounsaturated fats such as olive oil.

Fat and Cholesterol Go Together

The catch here is that few foods (except some shellfish and egg yolks) are high in saturated fat without also being high in cholesterol. This means that the most efficient way to lower blood cholesterol is to decrease the amount of saturated fat in your diet. You cannot reduce one without reducing the other at the same time.

Fat City: Making Your Way Through the Crowded Saturated and Polyunsaturated Pathways

It can be a maze of fats! Which way to turn? Which ones to avoid? Fat can be a detour or roadway in your search for a healthier and younger heart system. You can go in the right direction toward a longer lifeline, with a better understanding of the fat picture. Let's talk the language of these necessary and unnecessary "evils."

Cholesterol

A waxlike compound (sterol) found in all animal cells, including those of the human body; it is part of the cell membrane and a building block for bile salts and sex hormones. Produced by most body cells, but especially by the intestine and liver, it influences digestion because it is needed for bile production.

Dietary cholesterol. This is found only in animal foods and products such as meat, fish, poultry, and egg yolks and foods made from animal products.

Blood cholesterol. This is found in the blood and is strongly linked to risk and incidence of coronary heart disease. Eating too much cholesterol and saturated fat raises blood cholesterol levels, which causes cells to become overloaded in the blood vessel linings. This leads to atherosclerosis or hardening of the arteries. (Atherosclerosis refers to the clogging of blood vessels by deposits of cholesterol and other minerals which may lead to a heart attack or stroke or aggravate arterioscleoris, which is a thickening-hardening of the arteries.)

Fats

Saturated Fats. Found mostly in meat and dairy foods, saturated refers to chemical bonds; saturated fats contain more hydrogen atoms than do other types of fats. These are usually solid at room temperature. These fats are constituted chemically so that they cannot absorb additional hydrogen.

Polyunsaturated Fats. Found mostly in vegetable foods such as liquid oils; these fats consist of molecules that have one or more double bonds that are capable of absorbing more hydrogen. They are liquid at room temperature. Polyunsaturated fat helps to clear saturated fat from the body.

Monounsaturated Fats. These come from vegetable sources and contain one hydrogen atom less in their structure than saturated fats. This type of fat does not appear to raise total blood cholesterol levels. It may be as effective as polyunsaturated fats in reducing the levels. Sources include olive and peanut oils.

The Good Versus the Bad Cholesterol

When you stand at the crossroads of "fat city" and wonder which way to go, you need to know that there are three avenues to explore. One will lead to a younger heart. The other two could lead to a collision! Let's look in these directions.

High-Density Lipoprotein

HDL, as it is called, is the *good* fat. It is considered protective because it helps to remove cholesterol from your body.

Low-Density Lipoprotein

The most common type of fat, LDL, tends to pick up cholesterol and deposit it for storage in various cells throughout the body.

Very-Low-Density Lipoprotein

VLDL is an even more hazardous fat that can cause accumulations of more cholesterol than the LDL and can be responsible for a serious overload.

Make Your Selection with Nutritional Therapy

You will be giving your heart and circulatory system a new lease on life with increased amounts of HDLs through more polyunsaturated fats and fewer saturated fats. You will help protect yourself against a collision and pile-up of accumulated debris of cholesterol blockages. You can use nutritional therapy to go down the pathway of HDLs to reach your goal of a healthier and younger heart.

Go Slowly with Polyunsaturated Fat Increase

Caution: Granted, polyunsaturated fat will help clear the saturated fat from your blood and lower cholesterol levels, but you need to proceed with caution. Excessively high levels of polyunsaturated fats may work too powerfully and *reduce* HDLs—that protective fatty substance that acts as a cholesterol sweeper. So proceed slowly and within reason.

Simple Nutritional Therapy Goal

It takes 2 grams of polyunsaturated fat to counteract the effect of 1 gram of saturated fat on blood cholesterol. Therefore, decreasing saturated fat will have a greater impact than will increasing polyunsaturated fat. You can do it by changing your meal program to meet the percentages given in Chart 5-1.

Less Cholesterol = Less Heart Disease

For each 1 percent reduction in blood cholesterol levels, there is a 2 percent drop in the risk of developing heart disease. Furthermore, according to NIH researchers, even if you have had one heart attack, you will be protected against a recurrence if you control your diet. Your goal is to help wash out excessive cholesterol and protect against further pileup of this risky blood fat.

Chart 5-1: THE BALANCING ACT: Common Foods and Their Proportions of Saturated and Polyunsaturated Fats

Experts advise counting total fat calories and also watching the ratio between polyunsaturated fats (found largely in plant and vegetable sources) and saturated fat (mainly in animal products).

Since it takes 2 grams of polyunsaturated fat to counteract the effects of 1 gram of saturated fat, experts suggest you eat foods with a 2:1 ratio or better of polyunsaturated to saturated fat.

Food	% Total Calories From Fat	% Calories Saturated Fat	% Calories Polyunsaturated Fat	Polyunsaturated To Saturated Fat Ratio (Ideal = 2:1)
Cheddar cheese	74%	47%	2%	2:47
Swiss cheese	76	43	2	2:43
American cheese	75	47	2	2:47
Edam cheese	70	44	2	2:44
Creamed cottage cheese (regular)	39	25	1	1:25
1% fat	13	8	less than 1	less than 1:8
Whole milk	49	31	2	2:31
2% Milk	34.6	22	1	1:22
Skim milk	4.6	3	trace	trace:3
Nondairy creamer	58.5	54	trace	trace:54
Half and Half	80	50	2.9	2.9:50
Yogurt, lowfat	13	8	less than 1	less than 1:8
Ice cream, vanilla	48	30	2	2:30
Ice milk, vanilla	28	17	1	1:17
Sherbert, orange	13	8	less than 1	less than 1:8

Chart 5-1: *(continued)*

Food	% Total Calories From Fat	% Calories Saturated Fat	% Calories Polyunsaturated Fat	Polyunsaturated To Saturated Fat Ratio (Ideal = 2:1)
Peanut butter	78	14	26	26:14
Tofu (bean curd)	52	8	27	27:8
Bologna, beef	81.5	33.5	3	3:33.5
Beef hot dog	82	33.4	3	3:33.4
Chicken hot dog	68	19	14	14:19
Turkey breast (no skin)	5	1.6	1.3	1.3:1.6
Turkey leg	21	7	6.3	6.3:7
Chicken breast (roasted, no skin)	19.5	5.5	4.2	4.2:5.5
Roast beef (eye of round, lean and trimmed of fat)	34	14	1.4	1.4:14
Ground beef (Lean, well-done)	57	23.5	2.3	2.3:23.5
Tuna (in soybean oil)	37	10	7.7	7.7:10

Source: U. S. Department of Agriculture.

The Simple Oil That Helps to Clear
Away the Cholesterol Threat

Olive oil is a powerful monounsaturated oil that helps to control and wash away cholesterol in the blood. It protects against any accumulation of fatty deposits that might threaten to narrow the vessels, reduce blood flow to the heart, and pose a risk of cardiovascular disease.

Olive oil helps the HDLs to transport cholesterol from the body's tissues to the liver where it can be either converted for use by the body or processed for elimination. Furthermore, olive oil is a monounsaturate that has a more stable shelf life, so it does not go rancid nearly as fast as the polyunsaturates.

Nutritional Therapy

Use olive oil as part of a salad dressing, mixed with various herbs, every day. Use the same olive oil in cooking for any recipe that calls for oil. You will be supercharging your cholesterol-cleansing HDLs to give you a clean heart and a healthier body, too.

Fish Oils Will Cleanse Arteries and
Strengthen Your Heart

Eating fish and using fish oils several times a week may significantly reduce fatty accumulations on your arteries and make you less likely to risk heart disease.

New epidemiological studies show that there is a much lower incidence of atherosclerosis in some populations that eat larger amounts of cold-water fish and fish oils.

The protective effect appears to be in the oils which seem to prevent the formation of artery-blocking deposits much better than vegetable oils.

The Heart Benefits of Fish Oils

The secret of the fat washing and heart saving is the unusual ingredients found in fish oils: *eicosapentaenoic acid* (EPA) and *docosahexaenoic acid* (DHA), two long-chain fatty acids. There are also some amounts of vitamins A and E. Between 5 and 40 percent of the fat in seafood consists of these omega-3 fatty acids, as they are called. In contrast, polyunsaturated vegetable oils are rich in omega-6 fatty acids such as linoleic acid. (The number refers to the location of the first unsaturated bond in the fat. In the omega-3 fats, the bond occurs between the third and fourth carbon; in the omega-6 variety, it occurs between the sixth and seventh.)

What's the Difference?

Researchers suspect that omega-6 fatty acids predispose to substances that encourage platelets to stick together. But in omega-3 fatty acids, the platelets are kept cleansed, and there is less of a tendency to congeal. So it seems that the omega-3 fatty acids protect the platelets against clotting. These substances make the platelets less sticky, and this protects against the threat of atherosclerosis. This can be a lifesaver!

In brief, the more omega-3 you consume, the less likely you are at risk of heart disease.

Where to Find Omega-3

The leading sources would be cold-water fish (and their oils) such as salmon, mackerel, sardines, cod, halibut. You can hook into these heart-protecting sources of EPA and DHA by planning your meal program to include at least 6 to 8 ounces of seafood four or five times a week. Boost the action of cleansing HDLs by taking fish liver oils, 1 tablespoon every day. This bountiful catch from the sea may well foil cardiovascular disease.

WINS HEART BATTLE—HOOK, LINE, AND SINKER—WITH FISH OILS

An electrocardiogram showed that factory foreman Victor DeN. had a fluttering heart. Blood tests showed he had a risky cholesterol reading of 350 milligrams per deciliter. Dangerous! Life-threatening! And he was only 52 years of age! He asked his cardiologist for a diet program to help bring readings under control. He was put on a low-animal-fat and higher-polyunsaturated-fat menu. In four weeks, his reading was down to 320. Too slow, his cardiologist observed. Swifter and safer action was needed. The doctor then made a simple nutritional therapeutic prescription: eat seafood from salmon, mackerel, sardines, cod, halibut throughout the week. Use seafood as a replacement for animal products. Each day, take 2–3 tablespoons of fish liver oil with either citrus juice or with some herbs as part of a raw vegetable salad. Results? In seven days, his reading was a safer 210 milligrams. His new cardiogram showed a steady beat. His pressure, too, was stabilized. The fish oils had rescued him from the threat of atherosclerosis and heart trouble. Victor DeN. considers his seafood program to be a lifesaver that brought him to safety.

Say "No" to Three Items; Say "Yes" to a Healthier Heart System

Your nutritional program should be planned to avoid three items that can be deleterious to your heart and health. These are

1. *Salt.* Because it absorbs water, salt can cause edema, which is a threat to the health of your heart. *Avoid* salt either from the shaker or in cooked foods as well as in packaged products.

2. *Caffeine.* For some people, caffeine stimulates the central nervous system, makes the heart beat faster, stirs up the metabolism, and plays havoc with the blood vessels. It may widen some but choke others. It could cause heart flutters. *Avoid* caffeine whether in coffee, tea, soft drinks, medications, even some confections.

3. *Sugar.* It can cause the rise of a lesser known blood fat called triglycerides. Sugar seems to build up excessive amounts of this fat, and this could cause a heart risk. *Avoid* sugar from the shaker or in cooked foods. Read labels of all packaged products to see if sugar is contained—along with salt or caffeine. If in doubt, pass up the product.

You can help keep cholesterol and fat in check and your heart in better shape by eliminating these three "no-no" items from your food program.

Triglycerides—The Sneaky Blood Fat You Need to Control

Triglycerides is the technical term for fats and oils. Your body's fat stores are triglycerides. Although your bloostream always contains some triglycerides, if they are elevated, they may be implicated in atherosclerosis, the disease process that leads to heart disease.

Triglycerides are often upstaged by cholesterol. They do not take such a bad rap, but a high level of these lipids (fatty substances) in your blood should not be disregarded. True, there is no *direct* link to cardiovascular disease as there is with cholesterol, there is an indicator of risk. Triglycerides can be sneaky and if allowed to become overloaded, might cause problems.

Nutritional Therapy

It is believed that sugar tends to predispose accumulation of triglycerides. So will animal fats. Avoidance of sugar is one important step in controlling the levels of this blood fat. Moderate animal fat intake is another decisive step. Control caloric intake along with saturated fats. Eliminate alcohol. These factors can help keep triglycerides in check and give further protection against atherosclerosis and heart disease.

WOMAN OVERCOMES "HEREDITY" WITH NUTRITIONAL THERAPY

Joan Y. came from a family that had many heart problems. Her parents and two older sisters had such difficulties and faced a shorter life span. But Joan Y. resolved not to follow in their ill-fated footsteps. She consulted a clinical heart specialist who would use nutrition as the first line of defense against such difficulties. Joan Y. was put on a fat-controlled eating program. She was told to avoid salt, caffeine, sugar totally. Also, she would take 2 tablespoons of fish liver oil daily. Together with prescribed exercise, she resisted the risk factors of fatty deposits on and within her arteries. Her cholesterol level was a constant 175 milligrams per deciliter. Her heart was in tip-top shape. This simple program of fat control and saying "no" to salt, caffeine, and sugar, and taking 2 tablespoons of fish liver oil daily helped her remain heart-healthy...for her entire life! She had won against predictions that "heredity" would end her in the early forties. She celebrated her seventy-eighth birthday—hale and hearty!

Garlic—Relieves Chest Pains

The old-time remedy of using garlic to ease chest pains is an important part of the nutritional therapy program for a healthier heart.

Garlic eases plaque formation in arteries; it is a prime source of allicin, an active sulfur-containing compound that is changed into diallyldisulphide in the system; this helps to liquefy cholesterol deposits, loosen plaque, reduce lipid (fat) levels in the blood and liver, and improve the action of the heart. Garlic also improves the flow of oxygen into the bloodstream, thereby relieving chest pain associated with heart conditions. (Medically, the condition is called angina pectoris, in which the heart muscle receives an insufficient blood supply, causing pain in the chest and often in the left arm and shoulder.) It is garlic that may well help to dilate the blood vessels, allow a better exchange of oxygen, and relieve pain.

GARLIC AS HEART "MEDICINE"

Philip K. was troubled with recurring chest pains. He feared the use of nitroglycerine, which would dilate the blood vessels but would also cause dizziness, loss of some of his senses, nervous tremors, and gastrointestinal upset. He asked a homeopathic physician if a less risky treatment could be found. He was told to eat at least four garlic cloves daily, along with a fat-controlled and salt-free program. Philip K. chewed the cloves together with parsley to ease the strong scent, on a daily basis. In 11 days, his chest pains were gone. No longer did he awaken in the middle of the night, terrified, clutching his pain-filled chest, gasping for air. Now, he felt brand new, thanks to garlic. He even took a few cloves at night as his "sleeping medicine," so he could sleep well and awaken with hearty good health!

How to Feast High on a Low-Fat Food Program

You want to enjoy taste in your foods. You have a right to favor taboo fat. You can be satisfied with fatty good taste, but with these simple adjustments. They get the fat out of food, but leave behind the taste! (See Charts 5-2, 5-3, and 5-4 for guidelines.)

Meats

Select the leanest cuts. Avoid those with marbling. Grind lean beef at home to prepare hamburger. *Caution:* commercially ground hamburger contains about three times as much fat. Before cooking, cut away as much fat as possible. For example, the fat pads under the skin of poultry and game.

Panbroiling: Use a heavyweight pan. Do not add oil or fat. Add meat. Cover pan and broil over low heat, turning meat once or twice. After meat is cooked, turn up heat the get browning effect of a broiler. Drain off all fat drippings (see below). Fish and organ meats do not panbroil well, but you can poach them over low heat by adding skim milk or water. Season liquid with a small amount of lemon juice, vinegar, or a dry wine. Add herbs and spices to taste.

Fat-Free Broths, Gravies, and Sauces: If you chill drippings, drainings, and commercial sauces after cooking, the fat will rise to the surface and solidify for easy removal. To remove fat while broth is in original pan, skim ice cubes through it. To prepare brown gravy from fat-free broth, add 1

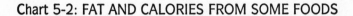

Chart 5-2: FAT AND CALORIES FROM SOME FOODS

If you choose to reduce the fat in your diet to 30 percent of your daily calories, for a 2,000-calorie diet that is about 67 grams of fat.

Food	Serving	Calories	Grams of Fat
Dairy Products			
Cheese			
American, pasteurized process	1 ounce	105	9
Cheddar	1 ounce	115	9
Cottage			
Creamed	½ cup	115	5
Low-fat (2%)	½ cup	100	2
Cream	1 ounce	100	10
Mozzarella, part skim	1 ounce		5
Parmesan	1 Tbsp	25	2
Swiss	1 ounce	105	8
Cream			
Half and half	2 Tbsp	40	3
Light, coffee, or table	2 Tbsp	60	6
Sour	2 Tbsp	50	5
Ice cream	1 cup	270	14
Ice milk	1 cup	185	6
Milk			
Whole	1 cup	150	8
Low-fat (2%)	1 cup	125	5
Nonfat, skim	1 cup	85	trace
Yogurt, low-fat, fruit-flavored	8 ounces	230	2
Meats			
Beef, coooked			
Braised or pot-roasted			
Less lean cuts, such as chuck blade, lean only	3 ounces	255	16
Leaner cuts, such as bottom round, lean only	3 ounces	190	8
Ground beef, broiled			
Lean	3 ounces	230	15
Regular	3 ounces	245	17

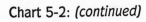

Chart 5-2: *(continued)*

Food	Serving	Calories	Grams of Fat
Roast, oven cooked			
Less lean cuts, such as rib, lean only	3 ounces	225	15
Leaner cuts, such as eye of round, lean only	3 ounces	155	6
Steak, sirloin, broiled			
Lean and fat	3 ounces	250	17
Lean	3 ounces	185	8
Lamb, cooked			
Chops, loin, broiled			
Lean and fat	3 ounces	250	17
Lean only	3 ounces	185	
Leg, roasted, lean only	3 ounces	160	7
Pork, cured, cooked			
Bacon, fried	3 slices	110	9
Ham, roasted			
Lean and fat	3 ounces	205	14
Lean only	3 ounces	135	5
Pork, fresh, cooked			
Chop, center loin			
Broiled			
Lean and fat	3 ounces	270	19
Lean only	3 ounces	195	9
Pan-fried			
Lean and fat	3 ounces	320	26
Lean only	3 ounces	225	14
Rib, roasted, lean only	3 ounces	210	12
Shoulder, braised, lean only	3 ounces	210	10
Spareribs, braised, lean and fat	3 ounces	340	26
Veal cutlet, braised or broiled	3 ounces	185	9
Sausages			
Bologna	2 ounces	180	16
Frankfurters	2 ounces (1 frank)	185	17

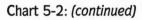

Chart 5-2: *(continued)*

Food	Serving	Calories	Grams of Fat
Pork, link or patty, cooked	2 ounces (4 links)	210	18
Salami, cooked type	2 ounces	145	11
Poultry Products			
Chicken			
Fried, flour-coated			
Dark meat with skin	3 ounces	240	14
Light meat with skin	3 ounces	210	10
Chicken, roasted			
Dark meat without skin	3 ounces	175	8
Light meat without skin	3 ounces	145	4
Duck, roasted, meat without skin	3 ounces	170	10
Turkey, roasted			
Dark meat without skin	3 ounces	160	6
Light meat without skin	3 ounces	135	3
Egg, hard cooked	1 large	80	6
Seafood			
Flounder, baked			
With butter or margarine	3 ounces	120	6
Without butter or margarine	3 ounces	85	1
Oysters, raw	3 ounces	55	2
Shrimp, French Fried	3 ounces	200	10
Shrimp, boiled or steamed	3 ounces	100	1
Tuna, packed in oil, drained	3 ounces	165	7
Tuna, packed in water, drained	3 ounces	135	1
Grain Products*			
Bread, white	1 slice	65	1
Biscuit, 2½ inches across	one	135	5
Muffin, plain, 2½ inches across	one	120	4
Pancake, 4 inches across	one	60	2
Other Foods			
Avocado	½	160	15
Butter, margarine	1 Tbsp	100	12

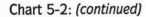

Chart 5-2: *(continued)*

Food	Serving	Calories	Grams of Fat
Cake, white layer, chocolate frosting	1 piece	265	11
Cookies, chocolate chip	4	185	11
Donut, yeast type, glazed	one	235	13
Mayonnaise	1 Tbsp	100	11
Oils	1 Tbsp	120	14
Peanut butter	1 Tbsp	95	8
Peanuts	½ cup	420	35
Salad dressing			
Regular	1 Tbsp	65	6
Low Calorie	1 Tbsp	20	1

*Most breads and cereals, dry beans and peas, and other vegetables and fruits (except avocados) contain only a trace of fat. However, spreads, fat, cream sauces, toppings, and dressings often added to these foods do contain fat.

Source: Human Nutrition Information Service, U.S. Department of Agriculture.

tablespoon of flour and one (salt-free) bouillon cube dissolved in ⅔ cup of water.

Browning Mushrooms and Onions

For better flavor, brown without fat by using just enough salt-free soy sauce or Worcestershire sauce to wet them. Cook in a covered pan over low heat.

Desserts

To make fruits without syrup tastier, add lemon juice, clove, or ginger. Since ½ cup of regular prepared gelatin has 70 calories, use dietetic gelatin and flavor with fruit or fruit juice.

Salad Oils and Dressings

Use polyunsaturated salad oils or margarine for seasoning, cooking, and baking instead of shortenings, butter, lard, and salt pork.

Chart 5-3: GUIDE TO REDUCING DIETARY FAT

This guide shows the amount of fat in diets with different proportions of calories from fat. For example, a 2,000-calorie diet calculated to have 30 percent of calories from fat has a total of 67 grams of fat or 600 calories from fat. Food labels can help you find how many grams of fat are contained in packaged foods.

Percentage of Calories Desired from Fat (%)	Total Calories From Fat Should Not Exceed (calories)	Total Grams of Fat Should Not Exceed (grams)
For a 1,500-calorie diet		
40	600	67
35	525	58
30	450	50
25	375	42
20	300	33
For a 2,000-calorie diet:		
40	800	89
35	700	78
30	600	67
25	500	56
20	400	44
For a 2,500-calorie diet:		
40	1,000	111
35	875	97
30	750	83
25	625	69
20	500	55

Chart 5-4: CHOLESTEROL CONTENT OF COMMON MEASURES OF SELECTED FOODS (in ascending order)

Food	Serving Size	Milligrams of Cholesterol
Milk, skim, fluid, or reconstituted dry	1 cup	5
Cottage cheese, uncreamed	½ cup	7
Lard	1 Tbsp	12
Cream, light table	1 fluid ounce	20
Cottage cheese, creamed	½ cup	24
Cream, half and half	¼ cup	26
Ice cream, regular, approximately 10% fat	½ cup	27
Cheese, cheddar	1 ounce	28
Milk, whole	1 cup	34
Butter	1 Tbsp	35
Oysters, salmon	3 ounces, cooked	40
Clams, halibut, tuna	3 ounces, cooked	55
Chicken, turkey, light meat	3 ounces, cooked	67
Beef, pork, lobster, chicken, turkey, dark meat	3 ounces, cooked	75
Lamb, veal, crab	3 ounces, cooked	85
Shrimp	3 ounces, cooked	130
Heart, beef	3 ounces, cooked	230
Egg	1 yolk or 1 egg	250
Liver, beef, calf, hog, lamb	3 ounces, cooked	370
Kidney	3 ounces, cooked	680
Brains	3 ounces, raw	1,700+

Source: "Cholesterol Content of Foods,"" R. M. Feeley, P. E. Criner, and B. K. Watt, *Journal of the American Dietitians Association*, Vol. 61 (1972), p. 134.

Low-Calorie "French" Dressing: Mix 1 cup of tomato juice and ¼ cup of apple cider vinegar or lemon juice. Add chopped onion, garlic, pepper, or any desired seasonings such as mustard, green pepper, celery seed, bay leaf, chili pepper, or Worcestershire or Tabasco sauce. For even lower calories, thin a mayonnaise-type dressing (not mayonnaise) with equal portions of apple cider vinegar or lemon juice and evaporated skim milk. Stir until smooth and let stand to thicken. Can be used on fruit, tuna salads, or cole slaw.

Low-Fat Whipped Cream: Mix 2 cups of evaporated skim milk with 1 teaspoon of lemon juice, or use 1½ cups of powdered skim milk reconstituted with ½ cup of water. Add a bit of honey. Chill and whip until thick.

"Creamed" Cottage Cheese: Add skim milk to dry cottage cheese and mix to get desired consistency. Cool overnight and flavor with buttermilk, spices, or vegetables when the curd is soft.

Sour Cream: To ½ cup plain "creamed" cottage cheese, add 1 tablespoon of apple cider vinegar or lemon juice. Blend or strain and beat mixture until fluffy. Add pepper, spices, or herbs, if desired.

Cream Soup

Use skim milk, dry skim milk, or water as recipe requires. Or thicken 1 cup of skim milk with 1 tablespoon of flour. You can also use the cooking water from boiled meats. Flavor with vegetables and add meats as allowed.

White Sauce

Thoroughly mix 1 tablespoon of flour in 1 cup of skim milk.

Egg Recipes

Substitute egg white for yolk in the following ratios: 1 egg white for 1 egg yolk, 2 egg whites for 1 whole egg, and 3 egg whites for 2 whole eggs.

Read Labels Carefully

Even low-cholesterol foods may have high amounts of saturated fats. A product may say that it contains "all" vegetable shortening. It may still have high saturated fat if it contains coconut or palm oils. Avoid these two "vegetable" oils. Hydrogenated vegetable oils are to be limited or avoided. Hydrogen is percolated back into these fats, transforming them from a polyunsaturated to saturated fat.

Oat Bran "Soaks Up" and "Dissolves" Cholesterol

Oat bran is a grain that is a rich source of dietary fiber, especially cellulose, hemicellulose, and pectin. It has been reported that this grain has the ability to "absorb" cholesterol and wash it out of the system. The reason is in its water-soluble properties. It acts like a sponge in absorbing the excess cholesterol and preparing it for elimination. If you enjoy a bowl of hot oat bran cereal several times a week, you may well be helping to keep cholesterol-fat levels under control. The mechanism is believed to be in oat bran's knack for binding bile acids in the intestines, breaking down cholesterol into more bile acids and helping to eliminate them. It is a natural way to keep your cholesterol in control.

The Spice That May Prevent a Blood Clot

You may be salt-restricted, but you can enjoy another tangy spice that is good for your heart! Meet capsicum or the familiar hot pepper. It contains an unusual ingredient that increases fibrinolytic activity that could well prevent thromboembolism (blood clot) among many people.

It is estimated that 8 out of 10 heart attacks are the result of development of blood clots on top of diseased blood vessels. Fibrinolytic action refers to clot-dissolving activity. A substance that can disolve the clot can save a life.

Capsicum is a prime source of a protein-substance that activates plasminogen, an item in the blood vessel walls that is needed to dissolve clots. It is capiscum that creates this process to activate the plasminogen to protect against vascular obstruction. You may consider it a built-in process to dissolve the threat of a heart attack.

Tangy Suggestion

Use a modest amount of capsicum in cooking as a seasoning to help maintain active levels of clot-dissolving plasminogen to keep your heart (and yourself) alive and healthy.

Take heart! Use nutritional therapy, along with better living habits such as exercise, stress reduction, emotional happiness, and you will give your heart its chance to live its maximum nine lives!

WRAP-UP

1. Keep your fat levels under control. Know the different types of fats and how some are helpful, others hurtful.
2. Slowly increase polyunsaturated fat intake at a 2:1 ratio over that of saturated fat to improve your heart's health.
3. Olive oil helps to control cholesterol in daily usage.
4. Fish oils can help you to win the battle against cholesterol.
5. Victor DeN. lowered cholesterol and stabilized heart health on a fish oil program.
6. Avoid salt, caffeine, and sugar, and you may well avoid a heart attack.
7. Be alert to triglycerides, a sneaky blood fat, boosted by sugar and animal fats as well as alcohol.
8. On a fat-controlled, fish oil program, Joan Y. celebrated her seventy-eighth birthday with a healthy heart; even when her parents and two older sisters had "inherited" cardiovascular disease.
9. Garlic is a natural chest pain antidote.
10. Philip K. used garlic to soothe his angina pain.
11. Oat bran is a spongelike cleanser of fat and cholesterol.
12. Capsicum, a hot pepper, may help to prevent a blood clot.

6

Allergic? Breathe Easier with Therapeutic Foods

Wheezing, sneezing, coughing, choking. These are the symptoms of an allergic attack. At work, at play, or in the middle of the night, the onset of such an attack can make you feel as if you're going to pass out. Until the frightening episode passes and you can breathe easier again, you feel that you have had a narrow escape. After all, life begins with breath; take away oxygen and you take away life! During an allergic attack, you have the terrifying fear that your breath of life will expire.

Allergy: What Is It?
Why Does It Happen?

An allergy is an unhealthy reaction to substances normally harmless. These may be taken into your body by being inhaled, by being swallowed, or by contact with the skin. Such sensitizing substances are called *allergens.* Common allergens include pollens, molds, house dust; animal danders (skin shed by dogs, cats, horses, rabbits); feathers (as in feather pillows); kapok, wool, dyes, chemicals used in industry; pollution; and medicines and insect stings, to name the most common.

How Allergen Triggers Attack

When the allergen is absorbed into your bloodstream, it stimulates certain small white blood cells (lymphocytes) to produce special substances known as allergic antibodies. These allergic antibodies react with the allergen and produce allergic inflammation and irritation in particularly sensitive areas of the body—the nose, eyes, lungs, digestive system.

This sensitivity may not be present at first contact with the allergen; it may develop after repeated exposure. *Example:* A new cat may not cause allergy until it has been living in a household for many months, and then the susceptible person becomes sensitized and develops a stuffy nose and sneezing or wheezing on further contact with the cat.

"Why Me? Why Does It Happen?"

This is asked when you find yourself allergic to substances that may not affect others in your midst. One answer is that your respiratory system may be malnourished so that offending substances are able to penetrate your bronchial breathing apparatus to cause distress. Your protective barrier has become fragile, your bronchial cells are easily invaded by irritants to cause the allergic reaction. The problem is compounded when antibodies attach themselves to certain cells—called mast cells—in the nasopharynx, lungs, lining of the body cavity, or the skin. When these mast cells become saturated with antibody complexes, a reaction takes place.

Histamine Is Released. This is a natural body substance that tells you an allergy attack is on the way. Histamine dilates your blood vessels, slows circulation, and lowers blood pressure; it causes runny eyes and nose, bronchial asthma, and headaches from dilation of blood vessels in the brain. Your levels of immunity have been reduced because of the bronchial fragility and the outpouring of an excess amount of histamine.

To help strengthen resistance to this sensitivity, certain foods and nutrition programs can act as "natural medicines" to rebuild your breathing apparatus and act as a fortress against allergic reactions.

How Beta-carotene Helps You to Win Battle Against Allergies

Beta-carotene is the predecessor of vitamin A, found in everyday fruits and vegetables. This preformed vitamin A is taken by your digestive system and is metabolized so that the retinols or molecules are transported to your bronchial tissues to strengthen and fortify the cells and tissues. Beta-carotene dispatches molecules to the critical points of your breathing segments, nourishing the walls and rebuilding the collagen, so that offending allergens are not able to penetrate easily. In effect, it is beta-carotene that will help give you immunity to allergies.

Beta-carotene Food Sources

Red, yellow, and dark green vegetables such as carrots, deep yellow squash, dark salad greens, sweet potato, broccoli are fine sources. Good fruit sources are the apricot, cantaloupe, peach, nectarine, and mango.

By boosting intake of these beta-carotene foods, you will be strengthening the mucous membranes of your respiratory system, building an inner fortress against the invasion of allergens; the same beta-carotene also buffers the outpouring of histamine which helps to ease and erase many of the symptomatic reactions of an allergy attack. In effect, beta-carotene is a form of natural therapy against allergies.

OVERCOMES "HEREDITY ALLERGY" IN THREE WEEKS WITH BETA-CAROTENE AS NUTRITIONAL THERAPY

The slightest dust would provoke a wheezing-choking attack in Walter G. until he would feel the breath of life being squeezed out of his chest. When the attack was over, he needed a half hour to recover and gasp precious air to replenish the lost supply. He was resigned to lifelong allergies because it "ran in the family." Because medications made him drowsy, caused headachelike side effects, as well as mental sluggishness, Walter G. decided to try an alternative treatment as suggested by a local nutritionist.

Walter G. was told to boost intake of beta-carotene foods. He switched to freshly prepared vegetable salads including greens, broccoli, yellow squash, and carrots. Desserts were always beta-carotene fruits such as cantaloupe, peaches, apricots.

Within ten days, he noticed he was becoming more resistant to offending dust or pollutants. By the fifteenth day, the beta-carotene program had so strengthened his breathing system so that he scarcely had an allergic attack when they were as common as twice a day, sometimes more. By the twenty-first day, Walter G. was completely free of allergic reactions. His medical nutritionist explained that the beta-carotene had rebuilt his fragile bronchial system so that offenders could not easily penetrate the tissues to cause distress.

Heredity? His nutritionist explained that allergies do run in the family but they can be controlled and corrected with therapy. Walter G. is now free of allergies, despite the heredity "theory," thanks to beta-carotene, which he calls his "natural allergy medicine."

Bioflavonoids Will Ease and Even Erase Allergic Episodes

Lesser known, but dynamically effective as an allergy fighter, are the family of substances known as bioflavonoids. These are natural ingredients found in specific foods, especially in the weblike inner netting of citrus fruits. Bioflavonoids are valuable in strengthening the permeability of capillaries so they resist invasion of irritating allergens. For many victims of allergies, bioflavonoids may well be the most powerful nutritional therapies needed to help ease and erase attacks.

Corrects Weakness, Strengthens Barriers

Bioflavonoids have the unique ability to increase capillary strength, regulate their permeability. There are millions of miles of tiny blood vessels, capillaries, that connect the arteries and veins in the tissues. Bioflavonoids work with vitamin C in keeping collagen, the intercellular cement in a healthy condition by correcting weaknesses and strengthening resistant barriers.

Bioflavonoids prevent breakage, so-called hemorrhages or ruptures in the capillaries and connective tissues, which might otherwise admit viral and bacterial infections. By correcting the disturbances in capillary permeability, by restoring strength and stability in the cells of the bronchial and entire respiratory tract, bioflavonoids become an effective therapy in the correction and prevention of allergic reactions.

How to Eat Your Way to Allergic Healing

Bioflavonoids are found in green peppers, citrus fruits, grapes, rose hips, apricots, black currants, acerola cherries, apricots, and strawberries. *Caution:* Because these allergy-fighting nutrients are water-soluble and heat-sensitive, these foods must be eaten *raw.* The bioflavonoids are largely destroyed by cooking or preserving.

Simple Nutritional Therapy Program

Keep a variety of the bioflavonoid foods in your refrigerator. Daily, especially in the morning when allergic resistance is low, have a platter of these various fruits. *Benefit:* Within moments, the bioflavonoids will exert prophylactic and therapeutic properties to boost the intercellular network of your breathing system so that offenders are resisted or "defused" to have much less distress.

Eat the Whole Fruit

Because bioflavonoids are so richly concentrated in the white pulp of the fruits and in the sheaths separating the sections in citrus, the whole fruit is your most potent source of a nutritional therapy. *Juices?* They are quick acting because they are concentrated, but when you squeeze the fruit, you leave most of the bioflavonoids in the peels. *Balance:* Emphasize whole fruits in the morning. Drink a glass of juice in the afternoon. Have a whole fruit in the evening to help build respiratory resistance so you are less likely to have a night attack. It is this balance that should form your basic nutritional therapy program against allergies.

FRUITS ARE MY ALLERGY MEDICINE

Antihistamines made Dorothy W. so dizzy she could hardly concentrate on her driving, let-alone exacting work at her video display terminal in the large corporation where she was employed. Yet she always insisted she was "hooked" on her drugs because without them, she would continuously erupt into choking spasms and hacking coughs without any advance warning. Her health and her job were both threatened. How could she free herself from the slavery of the medicines along with allergies?

The company nurse, also a dietician, suggested she try boosting bioflavonoid intake to build resistance from within. She provided a list of the proper fruits and recommended ample amounts on a daily basis. Dorothy W. felt she "had nothing to lose but the allergies," so she started enjoying the raw fruits.

Within six days, she felt better able to breathe. What triggered the choking attacks was less frequently pulled. Taking less medication, Dorothy W. still had fewer allergic reactions. By the end of the second week, she was able to do without her drugs and experience almost no symptoms. But when she discontinued the tasty bioflavonoid-rich fruits, she had itching, runny nose, constant sneezing, and coughing. Now she knew that the bioflavonoids were working. She eventually made a healthy changeover and took just the fruits as natural therapies. She could boast to family and coworkers that the fruits were her allergy medicines. They helped her become free of breathing disorders.

Garlic—The Quick-Acting Allergy Healer

A "wonder food" that has been found to possess nutritional and medicinal properties, garlic is a quick-acting allergy healer.

Garlic is known as being an antitoxin; that is, it defends and strengthens the body against allergens. It neutralizes toxins present in the system and "knocks out" their irritating threats to protect against respiratory attacks.

Garlic is a prime source of *allicin,* a substance that boosts the antibacterial and antiinflammatory reactions that help to improve your resistance against offending substances.

Natural Antibiotic

Garlic also contains *aliin,* a sulfur-rich amino acid from which *allicin* is made via the action of the enzyme *alliinase.* This creates a natural antibiotic effect to help neutralize and "weaken" the offender and prepare it for elimination.

Nutritional Therapy Power of Garlic

Garlic prevents allergic reactions because it stabilizes the nasal mast cells, thereby preventing the release of histamine and other symptom-producing substances into respiratory tract tissues. It has other nutritionally therapeutic advantages as well in that it has neither stimulative or sedative side effects. Garlic has traditionally been recognized as the natural therapeutic food to combat and heal allergic problems.

How to Breathe Easier with Garlic
Decongestant

If you are seeking an alternative to drugs, prepare this breath-restoring garlic decongestant:

Allergy-Ease Tonic

Into 2 cups of freshly boiled water, add 3 crushed garlic cloves and 1 teaspoon grated ginger root. Cover pot with a tight lid and let simmer about 2 more minutes. Remove from heat and place on heat-resistant and nonburning surface. Lift pot lid. Deeply inhale the steam for about 3 minutes. *Benefits:* The allicin substance in the garlic will combine with the pungent odor of the ginger root to help open up blocked respiratory channels. Within moments, the garlic will create a decongestant reaction so that you can breathe easier and better.

You can also fill a mug with the same brew. Add a squeeze of lemon or lime. A teaspoon of honey is optional. Sip while comfortably hot. This tangy Allergy-Ease Tonic will be a natural therapy that acts as a potent decongestant.

Concerned over allergic distress while away from home? Just fill a thermos with the Allergy-Ease Tonic and take along with you. Makes a refreshing "break" that helps you to relax and also strengthen resistance to allergic unrest.

The Vitamin That Helps to Free You from Allergies

Any number of medications contain varying amounts of one particular nutrient—vitamin C. Science has long known that this nutrient has a powerful therapeutic effect in building inner resistance against allergens.

Rebuilds Respiratory Tract

Vitamin C performs or assists in the formation and maintenance of capillary walls, aids in cementing body cells together and in strengthening the walls of blood vessels, and guards against allergic infection by stimulating formation of white blood cells to counteract their potential harm. Vitamin C is needed to form new tissue and regenerate existing tissue throughout the body, especially in the respiratory tract and breathing apparatus. This vitamin is able to control the spread of viral infections. By inhibiting viral spread, the allergic reaction is kept under control, and you can breathe easier and better.

Nutritional Therapy Sources of Vitamin C

The best sources are all citrus fruits. Additional sources include tomatoes, cabbage, raw leafy vegetables, strawberries, and melons. *Preserving vitamin C:* Water-soluble, it is easily destroyed by heat and exposure to air. If you must cook, use small amounts of water. Vegetables should not be cut into small pieces until ready for cooking because the more surface exposed to air, the greater is the destruction of vitamin C.

How to Use

Daily, boost your intake of citrus fruits, and use vegetables as part of a salad. Vitamin C is available as a supplement, and in reported studies, about 2,500 milligrams a day has been found effective in bringing allergies under control.

Control, Correct, Cast Out Allergies with "Breathe-Again Remedy"

For quick relief, try this "Breathe-Again Remedy" that goes to work so fast, you may very well say "goodbye" to your allergies almost at once.

How to Prepare

Combine the juice of 1 lemon, 1 minced garlic clove, ⅛ teaspoon of cayenne pepper, and 1,000 milligrams of vitamin C. (Crush a tablet.) Just sip slowly whenever you feel an allergic attack on the approach.

Benefits of "Breathe-Again Remedy"

The vitamin C and bioflavonoid of the lemon combine with the germicidal ingredients of the garlic clove, become activated by the concentrated vitamin C, and are amplified with the cayenne pepper. In moments, the toxins and allergens are "knocked out" and eliminated. You can breathe again. (If the remedy is a bit too potent, feel free to cut it by adding a little water or any desired herbal or caffeine-free tea.)

Within moments, you should be able to breathe easily. Over a short period of time, these nutrients help restructure your bronchial system, creating a form of inner immunity against allergens, and you should be able to cast out your disorder and breathe freely again.

Garlic Milk Frees You from Allergies

A tasty nutritional therapy that is prepared in minutes offers fast relief from breathing problems. But this therapy has another refreshing benefit. It offers hope for healing of your allergies so that you will be able to free yourself from such distress. It is simple garlic milk.

How to Prepare

Heat 1 cup of milk until very hot. Add 1 teaspoon of vegetable oil, 1 tablespoon of honey, 1 teaspoon of grated fresh garlic. Stir thoroughly until as well mixed as possible. Let it become comfortably warm.

When to Drink

About 2 hours before retiring, sip this garlic milk slowly. Spoon out any garlic bits and chew them before swallowing. You will experience an immediate opening of airwaves and unblocking of bronchial tubes. You will breathe so well, you should be able to enjoy a good night's sleep.

Benefits of Garlic Milk

The calcium has a soothing reaction; this is the relaxant that helps to ease muscular congestion in your chest. The calcium combined with the natural carbohydrates of the honey is made more palatable by the oil; joining with the antibacterial ingredients of the garlic, you have a combination that actually washes away bronchial irritants. The garlic milk will work almost at once. It is especially desirable as a nigthcap because it induces restful sleep and works to keep your bronchial tubes open so you breathe healthfully and are not upset by a sudden coughing spell. You wake up feeling free of allergies.

NUTRITION HEALS ALLERGIES OVERNIGHT

Larry V. was troubled with recurring respiratory attacks and asthmatic difficulties. Worse, they kept awakening him repeatedly throughout the night which weakened his overall condition. Medications so drugged him that he felt the aftereffects for half of the next day. He feared having a lifelong allergy problem. His allergy specialist noted his side effects to drugs, so suggested he try the garlic milk that had been recommended by a local nutritionist. Larry W. prepared the natural remedy and took a glass every night for six nights. By the seventh night, he was able to sleep peacefully without any allergic attack. By the end of the third week, he was so free of distress, he no longer needed medication and felt that the breath of life was restored, thanks to the garlic milk.

The Everyday Food That Opens up
Clogged Airways

An old-world tangy condiment has emerged as more than a modern taste perk for most main dishes and salads. It helps to send streams of welcome air throughout the nasopharynx-respiratory network, and you free yourself from that choking-sputtering-breathless torment of allergies.

What Is It?

Ordinary horseradish! Prepared from radish roots, spiced with vinegar, it is so pungent, all you need is about ¼ or (at the most) a ½ teaspoon atop a cracker or a celery stalk. That's all! Just chew thoroughly and swallow. In minutes, perhaps seconds, the volatile spices of the horseradish will send streams of refreshing oxygen throughout your entire airways. You'll enjoy huge gulpings of fresh air. You will be able to say goodbye to your allergies, thanks to the power of horseradish in being able to unclog, open up the choked airways.

Sniff or Eat for Instant Relief

If ever you feel a choking attack, reach for a little bottle of horseradish and take a whiff. In seconds, you breathe better. Otherwise, just dab ¼ teaspoon on a small cracker and eat. Again, within seconds, you have refreshing relief. *Suggestion:* Carry a small bottle with you for use in emergencies or when you are not at home. Horseradish is available in ready-to-carry bottles at almost any food store or supermarket.

How to Drink Away Your Allergies

One magic mineral has been found to be of tremendous value in helping to correct the cause of your allergies, namely, your sensitivity to outside substances. It is *potassium.* It is found in a richly concentrated amount in *apple cider vinegar.* Made from whole compressed apples, properly fermented, this product is a powerhouse of potassium.

This mineral is needed to help maintain the electrical and chemical balance between your tissue cells and your blood. Potassium directs a normal flow of nerve signals and muscle contractions. It also promotes energy release to protect you against a sluggish feeling caused by clogged cells and tissues.

How to Use

Just stir in 2 tablespoons of apple cider vinegar in a glass of water or vegetable juice. Add a bit of lemon juice, if desired, for a tangier taste. Stir vigorously. Sip slowly. In minutes, the concentrated potassium helps to correct the respiratory imbalance and detoxify your bronchial tubes so you have better resistance against allergens.

A Glass a Day Keeps an Allergic Attack Away

To strengthen your forces of immunity against allergy attacks, plan to drink just one glass of this vinegar tonic each day. Over a brief period of time, the mineral content will repair your bronchial cells and help to provide better breathing transportation and, it is hoped, freedom from allergies.

Avoid These Foods and Avoid Allergic Outbreaks

Certain foods are antagonistic to your respiratory system and would be best avoided. These include caffeine in any form, refined sugar, salt, and refined carbohydrates that tend to clog your bronchial and breathing networks. *Careful:* Avoid foods or beverages that are either too hot or too cold. Temperature extremes can also trigger allergic outbreaks. Strike the happy medium and you should have a happy breathing system.

Checklist of Possible Allergic Triggers

These offenders should be avoided to help build resistance to allergies: vapors from cleaning solvents, paint, paint thinner, liquid chlorine bleach; sprays from furniture polish, starch, cleaners, room deodorizers; spray deodorants, perfumes; hair sprays, talcum powder, scented cosmetics; cloth upholstered furniture, carpets, draperies that gather dust; brooms and dusters that raise dust; dirty filters on hot air furnaces and air conditioners that put dust into the air.

Avoid blasts of cold air, excessive humidity, smoke-filled rooms, overexertion, and emotional upset.

Give your total body a chance to build resistance to allergies and with the use of nutritional therapy, you may very well be able to breathe mountain-fresh air, no matter where you are—free of distress.

HIGHLIGHTS

1. Allergies often develop because of a bronchial weakness that can be corrected with nutritional therapy.

2. Beta-carotene containing foods rebuild fragile cells to create inner immunity against allergen invaders.

3. Walter G. overcame "heredity allergy" in three weeks on a simple beta-carotene food program. He was able to quit drugs in favor of nutritional therapy.

4. Soothe and relax allergic episodes with bioflavonoids that correct capillary weakness and strengthen barriers against irritants. Everyday fruits and vegetables offer this allergic fortress.

5. Dorothy W. avoided antihistamines and the dizziness that accompanied their ingestion. She switched to fruits that became her allergy medicines. They did more than ease distress. They cured her allergies.

6. Garlic is a natural antibacterial and anti-inflammatory food that helps heal allergies almost at once.

7. The Allergy-Ease Tonic frees you from distress, no matter where you are.

8. Vitamin C rebuilds your respiratory tract to block allergic attacks.

9. The Breathe Again Remedy works instantly in knocking out allergens.

10. Larry V. corrected allergies overnight with garlic milk.

11. Horseradish is an old-world remedy to help you breathe better.

12. Potassium is a powerhouse of allergy relief. Try the beverage described today and breathe better tomorrow. Or earlier!

7

Foods That Soothe Stress...in Minutes

Stress has been dubbed the malady of our modern times. It is surely taking its toll when we note that one out of every two visits to family doctors is prompted by stress-related symptoms. Based on national surveys, business costs of stress are estimated at close to $75 billion a year because of absenteeism, company medical expenses, and lost productivity, or over $750 for very worker.

Stress is known to be a major contributor, either directly or indirectly, to coronary heart disease, cancer, lung ailments, accidental injuries, cirrhosis of the liver, and suicide—six of the leading causes of death in the United States.

Stress also plays a role in aggravating such diverse conditions as diabetes, herpes, multiple sclerosis, allergies, and cardiovascular disorders, to name a few. It is a worrisome sign of the times that the three bestselling drugs in the country are an ulcer medication, a hypertension drug, and a tranquilizer.

Are You a Victim of the Stress Epidemic?

When you allow your body to get all revved up, but have no release for the stress, you could become victim of the "fight-or-flight" response. You bottle up your emotions and may not be able to adopt either of those reactions. Here is a checklist of symptoms that could indicate you are becoming a victim of stress overload:

Recurring headaches, dry mouth, overeating/undereating, chain smoking, indigestion, ulcers, stomach knots, butterflies in stomach, alcoholism/drug dependence, ready tears, hyperactivity/listlessness, leg wagging, proneness to errors, decreased productivity, clammy hands, fatigue/weariness, muscle spasms/tightness, talking too much too fast, stomach cramps, diarrhea/constipation, nervous cough, feeling "faint" and an attitude of being impatient under all circumstances. Did you answer "yes" to more than one? You're stressed.

Adapt to Stress and Live Healthier

Daily life calls for being able to adapt to the positive and the negative situations or changes around you. Whether it is fighting or running from physical dangers, losing something or someone of value, facing deadliness, meeting challenges throughout the day, waiting on a very long line, or being given some bad news, you have to adapt. Your degree of health and happiness, in large part, depends upon how successful you are in this adaptation.

How Nutritional Therapy Helps Keep You Cool, Calm, Collected

The sense of panic, however mild, primes your muscles, whips up your glands, accelerates your digestive system, and causes an outpouring of adrenaline among other hormones, as well as a nutritional upheaval. To help soothe your frazzled nerves, certain foods as well as minerals are able to help take the edge off your tension centers.

The Mineral That Works as a Natural Tranquilizer: Magnesium

When faced with stressful situations, reach for magnesium, and within moments, you should feel the balm of tranquility pour over your frazzled nerves. This oft-neglected mineral has the ability to strengthen your inner reserves against stress to shield you from the grating thrust of irritating situations and circumstances.

Magnesium Is Soothing

This mineral is needed to help regulate your heartbeat, soothe your muscular system to protect against spasm, lift your moods, and protect against feelings of depression and irritability. Magnesium is highly concentrated in your red blood cells where it serves to act as a stress shield to help keep you calm in the face of problems.

Boost Magnesium—Boost Calmness

In times of stress, magnesium tends to be leached out of your cells, shunted out of your body via eliminative channels. Magnesium depletion can make you dangerously stressful. To protect against this risk, boost your intake of magnesium so it is available to your red blood cells to help keep you cool, calm, and collected when facing daily challenges. Magnesium will also protect against the potentially dangerous condition of arrhythmia or irregular heartbeat. It works as a natural tranquilizer. And it's drugless!

Recommended Dietary Allowance

The RDA calls for 300 milligrams daily for nonpregnant women, 450 milligrams daily for pregnant women, and 350 milligrams daily for men. (Although dosages slightly above are considered safe, medical supervision is recommended when this limit is exceeded.) Are you getting enough? Minimal stress, whether some loud talking or a sudden noise, will cause a leaking out of your magnesium stores. A deficiency makes you tense. You become nervous. You need to replace the loss without delay to avoid the health risks of prolonged stress.

Quick Relief for Stress

Reach for some magnesium, instead of a tranquilizer. You will be using a safe, simple and speedily effective nutritional therapy to soothe your stress, in minutes.

Chew Nuts and Release Stress Within 10 Minutes

A handful of nuts can act as a natural antidote to stress. Whenever you feel stressed, take a handful of shelled nuts and chew thoroughly. (Avoid salted or roasted nuts, which are irritating and also disturbing to the nervous and cardiovascular systems.) Within a few moments, the richly concentrated source of magnesium will go to work in soothing the hyperirritability of your nerves and muscles, strengthen your muscles, stabilize your heartbeat, and make you feel calm and more relaxed.

Magnesium in Nuts

Putting it simply: 60 small peanuts gives you about 210 milligrams of magnesium. Or 40 cashew nuts gives you about 200 milligrams of magnesium. These nuts are powerhouses of highly concentrated magnesium, the "natural tranquilizer" that acts as a speedy antidote to stress. You can chew your way to relaxation in 10 minutes, the approximate time required for the magnesium to begin its balmlike coating of your nerves from the time you began chewing the nuts. The chewing activity, itself, helps you to feel more relaxed as you "work off" tension.

COOLS OFF BURNOUT, MELTS ANXIETY, SOOTHES NERVES WITH MAGNESIUM

Industrial designer Michael C. was faced with endless deadlines. He loved his work but last-minute changes, increasing conferences, dealing with endless people made him feel he had too much of a good thing. He was exhausted by noontime. He would even lose his temper and say things he later regretted. An orthomolecular physician who specialized in correcting specific molecules in the brain to provide a more healthful emotional environment recommended that he build resistance to stress with a boost of magnesium.

Michael C. was told to take a recommended 250 milligrams of magnesium each morning. At the same time, he was told to carry a small supply of salt-free, shelled, and unroasted peanuts and/or cashews. "Chew them as a snack throughout the day," was the medical directive. "You should feel less anxious and more relaxed in minutes," was the benefit described by the physician.

From the start, Michael C. felt his tensions evaporating. He looked forward to his work schedule, even overtime. He smiled more frequently. He had fewer nervous reactions. He became more tolerant. The magnesium worked in minutes to replenish the losses that were caused by stress responses from his work. He calls the magnesium, his "natural tranquilizer."

The Food That Works as a Natural Sedative: Tryptophan

A little-known amino acid or protein derivative is able to help melt stress and act as a natural sedative to give your body and mind a feeling of total relaxation. That amino acid is *tryptophan*, and it is found in rich concentrations in *milk*.

How Tryptophan Washes Away Daily Cares

This amino acid is taken up by your brain to then stimulate the release of a soothing tranquilizer known as *serotonin*. It is this substance that tends to coat your neurotransmitters, that is, the chemical messengers that carry signals from one nerve cell to the next and control all emotions, perceptions, and bodily functions. These neurotransmitters are responsible for just about everything you do and feel. Under stress, they respond by making you more sensitive and alert so you can effectively respond to the situation. They also make you so tense and high strung, you become stressful. It is serotonin that acts as a protector by controlling the vigor of these neurotransmitters. Serotonin envelops these messengers, keeps them in check, and corrals them to protect against runaway impulses.

It is tryptophan that initiates the manufacture of serotonin to then help wash away your daily cares by keeping you calm and more relaxed. Yes, you still do face daily stresses, but tryptophan via serotonin has made you more resistant so that you meet the challenges with strength and emotional tranquility. This amino acid is a natural antidepressant! It makes you feel glad all over!

FEELS GOOD IN BODY AND MIND WITH STRESS-MELTING TRYPTOPHAN

The slightest upset made Jennifer Z. fly into a rage. The 42-year-old mother of three children felt she could no longer cope with everyday chores, some as simple as having to wait on a short line at the local market. Jennifer Z. could feel herself heading for a nervous breakdown.

Taking tranquilizers resulted in side effects, not to mention erratic behavior and the fear of becoming an addict, so she had to stop this health and life risk. Desperate, she sought help from a neurologist who suggested she boost her blood levels of tryptophan to provoke production of serotonin to act as a natural tranquilizer. How? She was told to drink two glasses of warm milk every day. Skim milk was recommended to control calorie-fat intake. If she still felt raw nerves, increase to three glasses of warm milk throughout the day.

Jennifer Z. was willing to do anything to get herself back in the mainstream of daily living. Within two days, she no longer flew off the handle. By the fourth day, she was laughing even on a long line at the market or when faced with many bundles of laundry or a sink full of dishes. The reason is that the tryptophan of the milk sent forth a soothing supply of tranquilizing serotonin to make the formerly stress-struck housewife now feel happy and relaxed. She explains to others that when she sips the milk, it is her "sedative." The milk with its tryptophan-serotonin became her natural therapy.

Food Sources of Natural Sedatives

While 1 glass of milk contains about 100 milligrams of tryptophan, you can use other sources for your natural sedative: cheddar cheese—316 milligrams per 3½ ounces; oatmeal—183 milligrams per 3½ ounces; spaghetti—150 milligrams per 3½ ounces; codfish—164 milligrams per 3½ ounces; shredded wheat—136 milligrams per 3½ ounces. *Suggestion:* Include these foods in your daily eating program and feel yourself relax in the face of stress. You will help avoid anxiety, replacing exhaustion with ambition and feeling better in a matter of minutes. These foods are nutritional therapies that act as natural sedatives.

Relax Yourself with the Antistress Vitamin: Pantothenate

Any type of stress, from a traffic jam to jam spilled on your shirt, will cause an outpouring of adrenaline from your adrenal glands sitting astride the surface of your kidneys. It can also drain out your nerves to make you a victim of stress.

Stress will cause a decrease in some of the white blood cells that protect your body against infection. Constant wear and tear will also cause a spillage of a valuable vitamin along with the adrenaline, namely, *pantothenate.*

Its name is taken from the Greek word *pantothen,* meaning "from all sides," and it does live up to its name. This vitamin is able to control the biochemical processes to ensure protection against loss of those substances that you need to resist stress.

How Pantothenate Can Help You Let Go and Live Longer

This antistress vitamin is present and important to every cell of your body. It is intimately involved in stress because it is absolutely required to the smooth functioning of your adrenal glands. If there is a deficiency of pantothenate, your adrenal glands are unable to fulfill their needed "fight-or-flight" response. Your glands go "on strike," refuse to produce needed hormones. Now you are in stressful trouble. *Reason:* without adrenaline

96

and other important hormones, you cannot operate on all cylinders and are especially sensitive to any situation that causes stress. You react with this supersensitivity and can fly off the handle at the slightest provocation. This is typical if you are deficient in this antistress vitamin that can protect you "from all sides."

Sources of Antistress Vitamin

Whole grain products, including brown rice, wheat germ, peanuts, and rice bran, are excellent sources of pantothenate. Also include soybeans, salmon, and peanuts. *Emphasize fresh foods.* In refining products, pantothenate is reduced or even removed, so your antistress plan should concentrate on utilizing fresh whole grains or other products that have not been subjected to much processing. (In canning, about 35 percent may be lost.)

With pantothenate on a daily basis, you can help keep yourself insulated from stressful situations and react with a smile on your face and in your thoughts.

Super Source of Pantothenate

It's richly concentrated in brewer's yeast, a grain product that is a top source of almost all the important B-complex vitamins. In particular, just 1 tablespoon gives you about 1 milligram. An average of 4 milligrams daily is recommended for most folks. But to cope with stress, a higher amount may be needed to keep your adrenals in top hormone-producing shape. Brewer's or nutritional yeast is available at most health stores and many supermarkets. Use it sprinkled over salads or blenderized in a vegetable juice and feel your mood lift, your attitudes adjusting, your happiness on the increase.

FROM SUICIDE TO SERENITY IN 12 DAYS

Stella N. could no longer cope with daily tasks. She had such wide mood swings, she started to take tranquilizers. When their effect wore off, she took stronger doses. She felt so tense, she would cry for no apparent reason, lose her temper, become overanxious. Insomnia was a problem. Shouting rages made her a terror to live with. There was talk of having her confined in an institution because of these violent outbreaks and mood changes that were feared to cause self-destruction.

Her sister, a registered nurse, took action, recognized the side effects caused by ingesting tranquilizers, and boosted Stella N.'s intake of pantothenate. In particular, she saw that Stella N. would take close to 2 tablespoons of brewer's yeast in a glass or two of vegetable juice, every single day.

Immediately, the shouting outbursts subsided. She looked more relaxed. Stella N. was calmer, slept better, was more rational to live with. By the tenth day, she felt "back from the dead" as the pantothenate restored her mental stability. By the twelfth day, the jitters and stressful reactions were gone. Now, she could enjoy her busy daily life with a bright attitude. Suicide? It was part of her past she preferred to forget. She was the picture of serenity, thanks to the daily intake of pantothenate, the antistress vitamin.

Antistress Vitamin Tonic

In a glass of vegetable juice, add 1 tablespoon of brewer's yeast and squeeze of lemon juice, if desired. Blenderize or stir vigorously. Then sip slowly. Within moments, the rich concentrate of nerve-soothing B-complex vitamins and the very ample supply of pantothenate will befriend your adrenals, nudging them to release needed hormones to help you deal better with stresses, either physical or mental.

Daily Antistress Foods

Top sources of pantothenate include beef liver, chicken liver, raw broccoli, turkey (dark meat), peanuts, dried peas, chicken (dark meat), mushrooms, cashews, brown rice, and dark whole grain flours. *Suggestion:* Include lots of whole, uprocessed foods in your daily eating plan. A bowl of oatmeal sprinkled with a ¼ teaspoon brewer's yeast and wheat germ is a great antistress buffer.

If the stress in your life is getting you down, it's time you upped your intake of pantothenate, the antistress vitamin!

How Calcium Keeps You Calm

Feel uptight? Troubled with anxiety attacks? Something eating at your nerves? The reason could be a deficiency of calcium, the mineral that has been considered better than psychotherapy insofar as stress healing is concerned. This mineral is able to soothe your irritations, to give you an anxiety-free outlook so you can be friendly with your nerves.

The Nutritional Therapy of Calcium for Stress

Studies have shown that an excess of lactate (or lactic acid) in body chemistry is responsible for much anxiety, nervousness, irritability, fear, and tension. Calcium is able to neutralize the nerve-irritating lactate. Calcium enters into a chemical association with lactate, transforming it into calcium lactate and reducing its capacity to produce anxiety reactions.

Nutritionally, calcium ions reside at the ends of nerve cells (synapses) and maintain electrical connections and communication between nerve cells. In a healthy nervous system, calcium combines with lactic acid around the sensitive nerve endings, preventing the acid from irritating the nervous system. But if too much lactic acid is in your system, or you are deficient in calcium to perform a neutralizing role, the result is stress, tension, and anxiety.

How to Use Calcium to Defuse Lactic Acid and Keep Calm

Milk is a good and easily absorbed source of calcium. A glass or two will give an appreciable supply to help keep lactic acid from inducing stress. Other sources would include 1 ounce of Gruyère cheese for 300 milligrams, 1 ounce of cheddar cheese for 211 milligrams, or 1 cup of tofu (soybean curd) for about 300 milligrams. Your goal would be at least 1,000 milligrams daily so it is rather easy to get enough of this stress-easing mineral. *Tip:* instead of a coffee break, have a milk or cheese break with a fresh fruit (1 small orange has about 40–50 milligrams, plus vitamin C, which helps to speed up calcium assimilation), and you should feel cheered up in moments.

Simple Eating Tips for Healthier Nerves

Eliminate the use of salt, sugar, hard fats, chemically processed foods, refined carbohydrates, caffeine, synthetic foods. Maintain a regular eating schedule. Eat in a calm atmosphere. Emphasize the antistress foods and nutrients described here and help yourself say goodbye to stress and hello to a refreshingly happy daily mood.

Happiness, it is said, is like a butterfly. The more you chase it, the more it will elude you. But turn your attention to other things and it comes and softly sits on your shoulder. Do not chase happiness with tranquilizers or mood-changing chemicals. Instead, turn your attention to nutritional therapy, and before you know it, you will sense the butterfly of happiness sitting softly on your shoulder.

MAIN POINTS

1. Stress need not be painful given the existence of myriad foods and nutrients that help to keep you calm and relaxed in the midst of turmoil.
2. Try magnesium, the mineral that works as a natural tranquilizer.
3. Chew nuts and release stress within 10 minutes via magnesium intake.
4. Michael C. cooled burnout, melted anxiety, and soothed his nerves with magnesium within a short time.
5. Jennifer Z. used tryptophan to melt stress and gave up her tranquilizer drugs forever.
6. Relax with pantothenate, the antistress vitamin.
7. Stella N. was saved from suicide and given serenity in 12 days with pantothenate as found in brewer's yeast.
8. The Anti-Stress Vitamin Tonic helps you become calm in minutes.
9. Calcium is the "keep calm" mineral that corrects the root cause of stress, the natural way.

8

Osteoporosis: How Nutritional Therapy Can Protect You from This Bone Robber

One out of every four women reading this book faces the threat of osteoporosis. This "silent killer" is on the increase. Osteoporosis is silent because the clinical features are not detected until the woman is in her fifties or sixties, and even then it may show only minimal signs to warn the victim of the "creeping disease" that could be fatal.

What Is Osteoporosis?

It is an age-related disorder characterized by decreased bone mass and by dangerous increased susceptibility to fractures, in the absence of other recognizable cause of bone loss.

Osteoporosis is a condition affecting as many as 20 million individuals in the United States. Approximately 1.3 million fractures attributable to osteoporosis occur annually in people aged 45 and older. Among those people who live to be age 90, about 33 percent of women and about 17 percent of men will suffer a hip fracture, most of these due to osteoporosis. The cost of osteoporosis in the United States has been estimated at $3.8 billion annually.

Any Early Clinical Features? How Is Killer Detected?

An early sign of osteoporosis is loss of height; this occurs when weakened bones of the spine (vertebrae) become compressed. Later, as the vertebrae fracture and collapse, a curving of the spine (often called "dowager's hump) may occur.

Caution: Osteoporosis, however, usually goes unrecognized until the spine becomes noticeably curved or until a hip, wrist, or other bone breaks. *Danger:* A minor fall can result in a broken bone, or a hip bone may fracture causing the fall. Normally there is no pain until a fracture occurs. Vertebrae sometimes fracture during routine activities such as bending, lifting, or rising from a chair or bed.

Hip Fractures, Male and Female Victims

Hip fractures are an important manifestation of osteoporosis. The affected population tends to be older and the sex distribution more even than in the case of vertebral fractures. Acute complications—hospitalization, depression, and mechanical failure of the surgical procedure—are common. *Most patients fail to recover normal activity. The mortality rate within one year approaches 20 percent.*

Why Are the Bones Eaten Away?

Bones maintain themselves throughout life by a process known as remodeling, in which small amounts of old bones are removed and new bone is formed in its place. *Problem:* Beginning at about age 35, however, a little more bone is lost than is gained. (Bone density reaches its peak around age 35.) Bone mass decreases most rapidly in the three to seven years following menopause.

The Female Hormone Connection

After age 35, there is a slowing down in the production of *estrogen,* the female hormone. It is believed that this hormone is needed to help the body absorb calcium, a mineral that nourishes the trabecular bone which makes up the central core of bone tissue. As estrogen diminishes and comes to a halt after the menopause has been completed, there is a serious reduction in the body's ability to nourish the bones with average amounts of calcium. Osteoporosis, or fragile, brittle, and thinning bones, starts to take place.

Is Estrogen So Important?

Absolutely! Estrogen appears to aid the body in using calcium to firm new bone tissue. Theoretically, when estrogen is lost as during the postmenopausal stage of life, bone becomes more sensitive to a hormone called PTH (parathyroid hormone), which is a major stimulator of bone destruction. PTH affects the passage of calcium through the body's system. It would appear simple to replace estrogen with a synthetic hormone pill, but some research cautions that this presents a danger of inducing cancer. Since less calcium is absorbed with diminishing estrogen, the sensible solution would be to boost intake of calcium to make up the deficiency. This can be effective, even without estrogen.

Bones, Formation, Mineral Needs

Bone is made up of calcium and phosphorus crystals, imbedded in a matrix of protein fibers. The calcium gives the bone its strength and rigidity; the protein (collagen, mostly) makes the bone somewhat flexible. Also found in bone are potassium, magnesium, citrate, sodium, and fluoride. These minerals help to hold the calcium and phosphorus crystals together.

Bone is living tissue. It is constantly being broken down and reformed, like all tissue in the body. Bone formation is vital for growth, for repair of microscopic fractures that result from everyday stress, and for the replacement of worn-out bone.

How Your Skeleton Is Rebuilt

It begins with bone breakdown. Bone-absorbing cells called *osteoclasts* dig cavities in the inner surface of the bone—microscopic cavities with new bone cells. These cells begin the bone rebuilding process by first producing the collagen matrix. This is followed by a laying down of the calcium and phosphorus crystals within the matrix—a process called *bone mineralization*. Yearly, from 10 to 30 percent of your entire skeleton is remodeled in this way.

Beware of These Bone Robbers

In addition to the biological cause of bone thinning, the lessening of estrogen and calcium absorption, other "thieves" of the strength of your bones include the following:

Stress

Any form of stress can drain calcium reserves from the blood and skeleton. In women, who have smaller bone masses than men, there are the stresses of monthly tension, childbearing, injuries, and especially the change of life.

Inactivity

Exercise is believed to be the only preventive or therapeutic measure that not only halts bone loss but actually stimulates the formation of new bone. Like muscles, bones respond to stress by becoming bigger and stronger. And like muscles, they weaken and shrink if not used. Exercise also creates small electrical potentials in bone tissue that stimulate the growth of new bone. But if there is a period of inactivity, these processes slow down and calcium is drained out of the bones, accelerating the onset of osteoporosis.

Vitamin D Deficiency

Vitamin D is available primarily from the sun (produced by the ultraviolet irradiation of an inactive form of vitamin D in your skin) and in limited amounts from foods such as milk, fish, and eggs. Stored in the liver, vitamin D becomes activated to perform two calcium-boosting reactions: (1) it increases the absorption of calcium in the intestines, and (2) it increases the reabsorption of calcium through the kidneys. It is also needed to maintain a proper level of calcium in the blood. Any excess or deficiency can cause bone loss. That's right. You could also have too much of a good thing, so it is unwise to overload on vitamin D. Strike a balance and you protect against calcium loss.

Alcohol, Tobacco

Alcohol impairs calcium absorption through the intestines; it may interfere with the ability of the liver to activate vitamin D. Liver damage of many alcoholics is linked to rapid bone loss. There is some association between smoking and bone loss. The negative effects on bone appear to be related in part to the number of cigarettes smoked. For example, women who smoked half a pack each day were found to have more bone mass than those who smoked a whole pack; nonsmokers had greater bone mass than did smokers. For the sake of your bones, your very life, give up smoking! And while you're at it, give up alcohol, too. Cast out these bone robbers!

Caffeine: Thief of Bone Mass

There appears to be a connection between heavy caffeine intake and the loss of bone mass. In particular, if you consume a lot of coffee, tea, or soft drinks, a higher proportion of calcium is excreted in your urine, which means that less is being absorbed into your bones. Best to switch to caffeine-free beverages, for the sake of skeletal health.

Soft Drinks

The high phosphorus content in soft drinks can upset your delicate calcium-phosphorus balance and cause loss of the important bone-building mineral. To offset this negative effect, just steer clear of soft drinks, the biggest source of excessive phosphorus.

Aluminum-Containing Antacids

Many over-the-counter antacid products are high in aluminum and other chemicals that increase the loss of calcium by the body. They are also known for causing constipation, so it would be best to limit their use. Many alcoholics take antacids on a regular basis to soothe their stomachs; this combination can be destructive in terms of overall bone mass.

Diuretics

They promote the production of urine and are often prescribed for persons with high blood pressure. But calcium is also lost in the urine, and this means that it needs to be replaced via foods, calcium beverages, and supplements.

How Is Osteoporosis Diagnosed?

Most diagnostic methods are not definitive. Sophisticated tests, including radionuclide tracer methods, blood and urine calcium levels, and calcium balance determinations are not able to detect bone loss in early stages. *Problem:* conventional X rays cannot diagnose it until it's too late—*bone loss is invisible until about 35 percent of the mass has been lost*—hence its name of being the sneaky or invisible killer!

More Reliable Device Available

A newer method is that of the single photon absorptiometry method. It offers an acceptable method of precise and accurate determination of bone mineral content and bone width. A *densitometer* is sensitive enough to detect a 1 to 3 percent loss of bone and is especially accurate at the midpoint of the arm, an area which has a correlation with the total weight of the skeleton, the total amount of calcium in the body, and the amount of bone in the femur, or hip bone.

How Calcium Will Nip Bone Loss in the Bud

While osteoporosis may be a multifactorial process, with the use of calcium as early in life as possible, there should be less loss of bone mass.

The usual daily intake of elemental (that amount which is absorbed) calcium in the United States, about 500 milligrams, falls well below the recommended dietary allowance of 800 milligrams.

How Much to Take?

It seems likely that an increase in calcium intake to 1,000 to 1,500 milligrams a day beginning well before the menopause will reduce the incidence of osteoporosis in postmenopausal women.

Calcium Is Lifesaving

Basically, calcium is essential for muscle contraction, blood clotting, plus brain and nerve function. It is a key nutrient in the process of bone mineralization. Remember when your mother told you to drink milk for strong bones? This was sound advice. Milk contains calcium plus vitamin D, which is converted by the liver and kidneys into a substance called *calcitriol,* a hormone that aids in bone rebuilding or remodeling by regulating the body's calcium level. Calcitriol allows the intestines to absorb calcium from foods and prevents the kidneys from eliminating calcium in the urine. So you can understand the value of calcium as a lifesaver.

Had Your Calcium Today?

Your goal is to prevent osteoporosis by building strong bones before age 35. (The thief starts its robbing between ages 30 and 35.) But even after age 35, you can help slow down or *halt* further progression with a calcium-rich program. Each day, your goal is to consume about 1,000 milligrams of calcium. It is like putting funds in a bank. You are building insurance or reserves and drawing interest in the form of stronger bones. But you need to put in that 1,000 to 1,500 milligrams of calcium daily into your bone bank. That means *daily*!

SIMPLE CALCIUM TABLET EXTENDS WOMAN'S LIFE

She almost skidded on a slippery sidewalk. Miraculously, someone grabbed her before she could have had a nasty fall and broken her hip. Emma S. was so upset she went to her family physician for a checkup and something to "calm the nervous system." He noted she was somewhat frail, although only 50. He prescribed calcium tablets at 1,500 milligrams daily. This mineral would also calm her nervous system, but its greatest benefit was to help stop bone loss. Emma S. was developing just a slight spinal curvature or "dowager's hump" which was warning enough of fragile bones. Within several weeks, tests showed she had an abundant amount of calcium, and the risk of a hip fracture (2 out of every 10 patients who sustain hip fractures die within three months) became markedly reduced. A near brush with almost certain hospitalization and high risk of death alerted Emma S. to the need for calcium—a lifesaving mineral she takes daily.

Why Calcium Boosting Is More Important in Wintertime

Seasonal changes have been observed by researchers to point out the importance of speeding up calcium intake before, during, and after winter. Bone mass is lowest following the winter months, when there is least exposure to sunlight. Conversely, it is highest in the fall, suggesting that sunlight may play a lifesaving role in preventing weak bones.

Calcium together with vitamin D should be increased if you are heading into or are in the midst of or are just emerging from cold winter months. Other factors that influence this variation in bone mass include seasonal changes in physical activity and diet.

Warm Up Your Bones with Calcium

If you are facing a cold climate, just plan to boost calcium potency so that you maintain from 1,000 to 1,500 milligrams daily. Ask your nutritionist about supplements to make it easy to maintain these levels daily. You will help keep your bones alive and strong throughout the winter.

A SIMPLE PROGRAM PREVENTS FRAGILE BONES

Fran M. had a thorough examination by her physician. An X ray revealed that she was developing osteoporosis because of the thinning bones. Yet Fran M. had no pain, no symptoms. To nip this problem in the bud, the doctor said that Fran M. would need to boost calcium intake to 1,500 milligrams daily; this would strengthen her skeleton, which otherwise threatened to become so weak that any sudden strain, bump, or fall could trigger a fracture from which she might never recover, might never survive. Calcium was a lifesaver thrown to the needy woman!

Can You Get Too Much Calcium?

There is the fear that excess milk consumption could lead to calcium deposits and kidney stones. While it is true that a *very high* consumption of calcium can increase this risk, amounts under 2,000 milligrams daily have minimal, if any, risk. The exception is an individual who has a family history or previous history of kidney stones; that person may be absorbing much more calcium than the average person. Medical guidance is suggested.

Is Milk the Only Answer to Protecting Against Osteoporosis?

It would seem so, when you see that 1 quart of milk will give you close to 1,200 milligrams of calcium, whether whole or low-fat. But it can be tiresome to drink that amount, every single day. Some people are lactose intolerant and cannot digest milk. Others simply do not prefer its taste. But milk still is a good source. Chart 8-1 shows other calcium sources. How can you boost calcium consumption without really tasting (or knowing) of the added milk?

Chart 8-1: CHECKLIST OF CALCIUM-CONTAINING FOODS

Food	Serving Size	Milligrams of Calcium
Milk, whole	1 cup	291
Milk, low fat	1 cup	297
Milk, chocolate	1 cup	280
Milk, half and half	1 cup	254
Milk, evaporated, canned	1 cup	675
Egg nog commercial	1 cup	330
Yogurt (depending on flavor)	1 cup	343-415
Cheddar cheese	1 ounce	204
Parmesan cheese	1 ounce	390
Provolone cheese	1 ounce	214
Swiss cheese	1 ounce	272
Almonds	1 cup	304
Hazelnuts	1 cup	240
Kale	1 cup	206
Collards	1 cup	357
Sardines (canned)	3 ounces	372
Blue cheese	1 ounce	150
Cottage cheese	1 cup	130
Mozzarella cheese (whole milk)	1 ounce	163
Mozzarella cheese (part skim)	1 ounce	207
American cheese	1 ounce	174
Broccoli	1 stalk	158
Spinach	1 cup	167
Ice cream, regular	1 cup	176
Ice cream, soft	1 cup	237
Egg	1 egg	28
Cabbage	1 cup	44
Cream cheese	1 ounce	23
Beef, pork, poultry	3 ounces	10
Apples, bananas	1 medium	10
Grapefruit	½ medium	20
Potatoes	1 medium	14
Carrots	1 medium	27
Lettuce	¼ head	27

Try Nonfat Dry Milk Powder

Depending on the brand, 1 tablespoon gives you 52 milligrams of calcium. One cup of the powder gives you 832 milligrams. Try some of these calcium-boosting tips:

- To increase milk's calcium content, just add 1 or 2 tablespoons of nonfat dry milk powder to every glass of fluid milk.
- Top a serving of cooked cereal with 2 tablespoons of the powder.
- Add up to 3 tablespoons of the powder to 1 cup of yogurt for a more robust flavor and more calcium.
- Get creamier and richer-tasting salad dressings when you combine 3 tablespoons of nonfat dry milk with 1 cup of your favorite creamy-style salad dressing.
- Stir ½ cup of nonfat dry milk into one 10 ¾ ounce can of undiluted cream soup; then add liquid milk to the soup base and heat as directed.
- Onion dips or any of your favorite cream-based dips can be boosted with calcium. Just add 3 tablespoons of nonfat dry milk to 1 cup of cream dip mixture.
- Blenderize nonfat dry milk and yogurt with your favorite fruit, water, and ice for a refreshing and calcium-enriched beverage.
- You use mayonnaise in so many things. Boost it with calcium. Just blend 2 tablespoons of nonfat dry milk into each ½ cup of mayonnaise. Your salad dressings, dip mixes, and sandwich spreads will help you reach your daily calcium goals.
- Mashed potatoes, anyone? Increase their calcium content by adding 2 tablespoons of nonfat dry milk to every cup of potatoes.
- Enrich those biscuits and yeast breads with calcium. To a biscuit recipe calling for 2 cups of flour, add ⅓ cup of nonfat dry milk. *Tip:* Add up to ¾ cup of the powder to a yeast bread recipe calling for 6 cups of flour.
- Cream or cheese sauces made using nonfat dry milk may be used in casseroles for a tasty and easy calcium-boosting dinner idea.
- Calcium absorption increase if this mineral is eaten with foods high in vitamin C (tomatoes, citrus fruits, green vegetables), so add more of these vitamin C foods to your salads and soups.

• Vitamin D, which is produced in the skin by the sun's rays, increases calcium absorption by your body. Vitamin D is almost always added to nonfat dry milk (read labels, please) so you needn't rely on sunshine, especially if you have been cautioned against excessive sun exposure.

Selecting a Calcium Supplement

Select one that is labeled as being *calcium carbonate* because it has the highest potency and absorption rate. Next you may want calcium lactate (unless you are lactose intolerant), calcium gluconate, and oyster shell (basically calcium carbonate). You can buy them in tablet, capsule, powder, or liquid form. Calcium, like other mineral nutrients, always comes in combination with other elements because, alone, minerals cannot be absorbed. Read labels, and select a *calcium carbonate* (prime choice) that has other minerals, too. This would be the easy way to take your 1,000 or 1,500 milligram dose daily.

Remember, your body needs and uses calcium every day. If it isn't getting what it needs from your diet, it will take it from the only other available source: your bones. With age, this deterioration can cause bones to break spontaneously, without impact. And can lead to stooped posture and shorter stature characteristically associated with old age.

Did you know that almost 20 percent of your body calcium is used up each year? It must be replaced by dietary or supplemental calcium. Protect yourself against osteoporosis and other threatening risks with adequate calcium in your food program. It is the simpler form of nutritional therapy that can be a lifesaver!

IN REVIEW

1. The silent killer of osteoporosis has no symptoms. It claims countless tens of thousands of lives and strikes women over the age of 45.

2. Note checklist of bone robbers and make a change in your life-style to ease stress, become more active, correct vitamin D intake, give up alcohol, tobacco, caffeine, soft drinks, aluminum, dangerous diuretics.

3. Plan to consume from 1,000 to 1,500 milligrams of calcium daily as insurance against bone theft.

4. Calcium is able to nip bone loss in the bud.

5. Emma S. had a near-accident that alerted her doctor to the need for calcium boosting which saved her life in the future.

6. Select a variety of calcium foods from the accompanying listing.

7. Boost calcium as cold weather approaches for better bone health.

8. Try the tasty and bone-strengthening nonfat dry milk powder tips to boost calcium intake, without really knowing it.

9. Fran M. had a routine test that detected the onset of bone loss and discovered how calcium could be a lifesaver. She was saved in time from the sneaky, silent, epidemic killer—osteoporosis!

9

How to Feed Your Brain a Youthful Memory

Troubled with memory lapses? Finding it difficult to remember names and faces? Cannot recall events that happened as recently as a few weeks ago? You may have a nutritional deficiency in your brain. Your memory banks need a few brain boosters found in everyday foods. With proper nutrition, you should be able to think more clearly and remember with more youthful alertness, no matter what your age. You *can* feed your brain a youthful memory.

The Human Computer

In your brain are 10 billion or more *neurons* (nerve cells) that perform the complex task of creating, storing, and retrieving knowledge. Chemical messengers or *neurotransmitters* pass from one neuron to another. The typical neurotransmitter has just told you what these words mean.

Miracle Neurotransmitters: Key to Brain Power

Memory, learning, brightness, being able to remember either simple or complex matters are all determined by neurotransmitters. They are charged with the responsibility of carrying messages between neurons. These messengers control more than IQ. They help you sleep, they wake you up, they make you happy or sad, tense or calm. They influence your appetite, your dreams, your activities. You cannot make a move without neurotransmitters—they control your coordination, too. They are miracles in the sense that they are at the helm of every movement made by your body or mind.

How Your Brain Stays Young

In a state of arousal, your brain is primed to respond quickly to external stimuli. Specifically, the neurotransmitters *norepinephrine (nor-*

adrenalin) and *acetylcholine* keep some brain cells primed to "fire" in response to stimulation. There is strong evidence that acetylcholine is involved in memory. This chemical messenger is sent to the *cerebral cortex,* the furrowed outer surface of the largest and most highly evolved part of the brain, the *cerebrum.* An acetylcholine factory, called the *nucleus basalis,* is located at the base of the cerebrum. When neurons in this region fire, they release acetylcholine that binds to receptors on target cells in the cerebral cortex. Activation of the *hippocampus,* a finger-sized bundle of neural tissue deep within the cerebrum, helps your memory stay young. The hippocampus works like a telephone switchboard, connecting various cortical areas with the new fact in a find of "conference call."

Eventually, these cortical areas learn to "dial direct"; that is, they establish independent neural connections called *circuits* among themselves. And the new memory is said to be consolidated. With a supply of nutrients that stimulate the release of acetylcholine, your brain is able to stay young and alert.

Alzheimer's Disease May Be Nutritional Deficiency

What Is Alzheimer's Disease?

Alzheimer's disease is a disorder that affects the cells of the brain. It causes intellectual impairment, also known as senile dementia. It first affects the memory, and then the personality. As the disease progresses, protein threads in nerve cells of the brain become twisted around each other into tangles; some pieces of degenerating nerve cells become disarranged. The more formations, the worse the symptoms. In particular, there is a form of molecular starvation. Under microscope, these changes appear as a tangle of neurofibrillary fibers.

The Nutritional Connection

There is a serious reduction—as much as 90 percent—in a particular brain protein or enzyme (choline acetyltransferase) that is involved in the passage of nerve signals. It is this deficiency that causes a sluggishness and slowing of the production of acetylcholine, the chemical compound active in transmission of nerve impulses. With a boosting of choline, there is a subsequent increase in the production of neurotransmitters that help keep your brain and memory in youthful vitality.

Choline: The Brain-Boosting Nutrient
That Helps You Think Young

Choline is an essential nutrient that is needed to form acetylcholine, the neurotransmitter that helps keep your memory alert and your thinking processes in a youthful condition.

Choline Prevents Brain Aging

Normally, the brain cells wear out; the membranes become more rigid with fatty deposits and lose their ability to take in and release brain chemicals to relay messages. This can cause memory loss and confused thinking. But it is choline that seems to repress or delay this membrane hardening.

Further, if the brain cells are seriously deficient in choline, they lose dendritic spines, the chemical receptor areas needed to pass along information. Having too few dendritic spines is like having a poor telephone connection. Messages are distorted and lost.

Choline to the Rescue

It is choline that is able to help keep the protein threads from becoming what are known as *neurofibrillary tangles.* Choline acts as a supervisor to see that everything moves smoothly and in proper order. Choline also protects against one major contributory cause of Alzheimer's disease, namely, *neuritic plaques.* These are pairs of fine nerve fibers twisted around each other and lying in the cell bodies of neurons. The greater the number of tangles and plaques, the greater the severity of the symptoms of brain weakness and memory loss and approaching senility. It is choline that prevents the rapid breakdown so that the transmitter is coaxed into working with more vigor and health. This brain-boosting nutrient has the ability to help create the process that keeps your thinking apparatus in a youthful condition.

Where to Find Brain-Boosting Choline

Natural food sources include egg yolks, brain, heart, green leafy vegetables, legumes, brewer's yeast, liver, and wheat germ. The richest source is found in *lecithin,* a soybean product, that is available as granules or in tablet form. It may be preferable to the high-fat or high-cholesterol animal sources just listed. With lecithin, the choline is speedily absorbed by your body. It then maintains a form of "law and order" in your brain to protect against fiber tangles and nerve plaques so that you are guarded against so-called senility. Choline also increases acetylcholine to keep your neurotransmitters moving along swiftly so you have an active and alert brain. You can think young with choline!

FROM "MISSING MARBLES" TO "SUPERSMART" IN 21 DAYS

Building supervisor Alex Q. kept forgetting schedules. His memory had so many gaps, he neglected setting certain switches throughout the foundry, resulting in near disaster one morning. A long-time satisfactory worker for the sprawling manufacturing plant, Alex Q. was said to be developing Alzheimer's or senility. Was he doomed at the young age of 56? Not according to a psychiatrist who used nutrition as part of therapy. He made a simple dietary correction in Alex Q.'s food program. Daily, Alex was to take 4 heaping tablespoons of lecithin granules in a beverage, sprinkled over his salad, cereal, or baked in a casserole or entree, even in a soup. Just 4 tablespoons daily.

Results? Within 11 days, his "missing marbles" as coworkers unkindly whispered behind his back, were now "found" and "returned." By the end of the eighteenth day, Alex Q. had a razor sharp memory, better than ever before. By the twenty-first day, he was "supersmart" and could fulfill daily responsibilities without even referring to a written list. He had a terrific power of total recall. Just give him a list of duties and he could perform them without any note taking. Now his coworkers look upon him as the "big brain." It was choline in lecithin that saved him from senility and gave him a super memory power!

How to Boost Brain Power with Choline Therapy

On a daily basis, make choline available to help put youthful life into your neurotransmitters. Remember, memory is formed with the use of acetylcholine, and it is the nutrient, choline, that prompts the manufacture of this brain booster. To have choline available, try these easy (and tasty) nutritional therapies.

Brain Tonic

Add 4 tablespoons of lecithin granules to a tall glass filled with diced green vegetables; stir in ¼ teaspoon brewer's yeast and 1 tablespoon wheat germ. Add a small amount of water or any salt-free vegetable juice.

Blenderize until thoroughly assimilated, about 3 minutes. Drink slowly. *Tip:* Give your brain a special boost by drinking this tonic about two hours after breakfast. You'll feel mental vigor almost from the start. This Brain Tonic is a richly concentrated powerhouse of choline that works quickly and lasts throughout the day.

Brain Spice

Fill a salt shaker with lecithin. Use it to sprinkle soups, salads, main dishes, throughout your eating program. You will be giving your brain day-long choline to help keep you thinking with youthful alertness. If anyone asks what you are seasoning your food with, explain that it is your Brain Spice!

Brain Food

Just add 1 or 2 tablespoons of lecithin to any baked dish. It especially blends in with vegetable or meatloaf recipes. It is also good in soups, stews, and casseroles. Whenever you prepare your recipe, just remember to add the Brain Food and you'll soon have no fear of losing that memory gift!

Lecithin is available in most health food stores and special diet sections of larger food markets.

Think Better with Tryptophan

Tryptophan, an essential amino acid, is required for the formation of serotonin, a neurotransmitter that helps to control your emotions, pain levels, and sleep. It is tryptophan that is intimately involved in sparking the release of those valuable neurotransmitters that help you to think and act with more vigor.

How Tryptophan Is a Brain Booster

This amino acid is converted into a variety of intermediate compounds flowing into nicotinamide adenine dinucleotide (NAD) or into another variety of substances flowing into serotonin. Serotonin helps the brain to sort out the confusion, protect against the tangling of filaments, and improve the route of the neurotransmitters to ensure clearer thinking. Tryptophan also helps your brain to relax and, in many cases, helps you to sleep much better at night.

Think Better, Become Alert, Feel Happier

Tryptophan releases serotonin, which, as you know, can improve your ability to think better, alleviate depression, and diminish your sensitivity to negative stimuli. It is the tryptophan-dispatched serotonin that acts as a natural mood regulator and dispels depression. You become happier and can function with more vitality. It is tryptophan that helps you feel glad all over.

Where to Find Tryptophan

It is abundant in milk, cheese, most meat products, and egg yolk. You will also find it in supplement form at most health stores.

FROM "MEMORY LAPSES" TO "COMPUTER BRAIN" AT AGE 63

His family and friends felt embarrassed over the way Mark D. kept forgetting dates, special events, even names of familiar faces. Frequently, he was discovered to be staring into space. Questions had to be repeated and the answers were vague. Mark D. had always been an active industrial executive, so this constant forgetfulness and the "memory lapses" began to worry those in his surroundings.

When he forgot to lock the front door and, worse, got into his car and drove for 5 minutes without knowing where he was going, the family decided something had to be done.

Senile? A physician who specialized in the relationship of nutritional failures to physiological dysfunction diagnosed the condition as a deficiency in specific elements. The physician recommended boosting tryptophan intake to a prescribed 1,000 milligrams per day. He also prescribed 250 milligrams of choline per day. The purpose was to activate neurotransmitters so neurons would reach into many areas of the brain, including the hippocampus.

Within 12 days, Mark D. was completely remade. He had a rapid-fire memory again; his thinking was so sharp, he could repeat sentences, even paragraphs, to prove he had superretentive ability. He was no longer the victim of deficiency-caused "memory lapses" but had a "computer brain" at his young age of 63.

It was the combination of tryptophan and choline that protected him from the risk of so-called senility. This nutritional therapy gave him a "computer brain."

How to Wake up Your "Tired Brain" with Tyrosine

Can't remember names or faces? Need to ask someone to repeat some simple information? Is your mind a blank? The reason could be a deficiency in tyrosine, an amino acid found in most dairy products, eggs, and animal foods. Tyrosine could help fill in the blank spots in your memory bank.

How to Think Better with Tyrosine

A number of neurotransmitters or chemical messengers originate from tyrosine which prompts the transmission of vital facts along your set of neurons or brain cells. It is tyrosine that is one of the valuable nutrients that acts as a stimulus to the cell body to prompt the electrical impulses to continue on their course.

Tyrosine is transformed into noraderenaline, which is then converted into adrenaline, which is needed to prompt your brain into thinking action. It is this amino acid that influences the production and concentration of the valuable chemical messengers that help you to think and remember better. Tyrosine is an important influence on your brain receptors, giving you the ability to understand, utilize, and store information in your memory bank.

Sources of Tyrosine

Tyrosine is found in dairy foods, cheeses, egg yolk, and most animal foods. It is also available as a food supplement from your health store.

NO LONGER CONFUSED, MEMORY BECOMES KEEN,
FEELS "ALIVE" AGAIN

Louise O'L. was a private secretary in a large grain corporation. Coworkers and superiors noticed she frequently forgot to pass along messages. If notes were written, she could not remember where she had placed them. Although she was not even 52, she displayed symptoms of senility; worse, Alzheimer's. Was she to be pitied or helped?

The corporation physician suggested that Louise O'L. boost her increase of brain-stimulating foods, especially tyrosine. In particular, tyrosine would initiate the production of the valuable neurotransmitters involved in both learning and memory. It would nourish the hippocampus by strengthening and regenerating the bundle of neural tissue deep within the cerebrum segment of the brain.

Louise O'L. took prescribed potencies of tyrosine. Within one week, she was able to "straighten" her formerly confused thoughts. Her memory was keen and now she felt "alive" because she happily exclaimed, "I have my head together!" Not only was her job saved, but she was given a promotion and salary increase because her tyrosine-stimulated brain made her all the better as a valued employee!

Tyrosine in the Morning, Better Thinking Within One Hour

This amino acid is unique in it works very swiftly. It envelopes the nerve cells that manufacture acetylcholine and improves their functions to stimulate thinking. *Suggestion:* take a tyrosine supplement in the morning for better absorption benefit. Reward: within 30 minutes, the tyrosine offers a form of protection to guard against the breakdown of the neurotransmitters and prolong their action. For so-called "supermemory" or "thinking-plus power," try a tyrosine supplement in the morning. You will have a terrific "brain-booster" reaction within an hour and enjoy long-lasting thinking ability.

How to Rejuvenate Your Thinking Abilities

You can increase your brain power by following some everyday programs to put new life into your neurotransmitters.

Correct Your Posture

Slumped over? You could be putting a crimp on the oxygen-carrying blood supply to your brain. If you let your head hang over your chest and your chin jut out, you are squeezing arteries passing through the spinal columns to your brain. Penalty? Fuzzy thinking, forgetfulness—even if you are young! Hunched-over posture can shortchange the supply of iron to your red blood cells and impair your memory. Iron is richly concentrated in the reticular activating system of your brain that keeps you mentally alert. So maintain good posture. Let oxygen pour into your brain along with iron-rich blood (your brain needs up to 30 times more blood than any other body organ) and "think young"!

Avoid Aluminum in Any Form

Believed to be a possible destroyer of nerve cells, aluminum has been found in dangerously high amounts in the brains of victims of Alzheimer's. The metal shows up in cells that also contain neurofibrillary tangles. Whether aluminum deposits cause memory destruction by acting as a toxin, or whether the metal accumulates as a result of other biological changes is not known. But it would make good sense to avoid aluminum. It is found in any number of patent remedies such as antacids and over-the-counter as well as prescribed medications. Check labels. Ask your pharmacist and/or physician. Keep your brain free of aluminum and you may well keep it alive, longer.

Straighten out your thinking by using nutritional therapy to keep the protein threads of your brain in smooth and untangled working order. With the use of nutrition, you will help to boost your thinking powers, protect against the threat of senility or Alzheimer's, and enrich your life!

POINTS TO REMEMBER

1. Your brain stays young with the use of nutritional therapy to feed certain segments and initiate processes to help you think better.

2. Choline is a brain-boosting nutrient that helps fill in the gaps in your memory.

3. Alex Q. corrected his "missing marbles" and became "supersmart" within 21 days by using choline in lecithin, a soybean food product available in all health stores.

4. Improve mental powers with the Brain Tonic, the Brain Spice, and the Brain Food in your daily eating plan.

5. Think better with brain-boosting tryptophan, a miracle amino acid.

6. Mark D. went from "memory lapses" to a "computer brain" by using this supplement. He was a young 63 with this nutrient.

7. Tyrosine helps you think better, almost immediately. Louise O'L. corrected confusion, sharpened her memory, and was "restored to life" with the use of this brain-boosting nutrient.

8. Improve your brain powers with corrected posture and avoiding aluminum.

—»»———— 10 ————«—

Healing Digestive Disorders with Soothing Foods

One American in ten is troubled with chronic digestive disease. One in two suffers from occasional digestive distress. Disorders of the digestive tract are responsible for $50 billion annually in lost work, lost wages, and disability and health care payments. Every day, 200,000 people stay home from work because of an illness associated with the digestive tract. More people are hospitalized with disorders of the digestive system, or gastrointestinal tract (GI tract), than with any other group of disorders. More seriously, digestive diseases are responsible for approximately 200,000 deaths each year.

Yet, based on a survey, 66 percent of those queried admitted knowing "only a little" or "nothing at all" about digestive disorders.[1] Small wonder the problem is striking more and more people, particularly those in the middle years, after years of disregard and abuse of this gateway system to your total well-being.

Why Does Your Digestive System Cry Out with Rage?

Expect trouble when you tell your stomach, "Just one more bit" or else "I'll try to eat the whole thing" or "I know I'll regret it but that second helping looks too good to resist."

Next morning (or sooner), your digestive system protests in the form of cramps, bloating, nausea, and diarrhea that may continue for a day or two or more before the grumbles finally go away. Symptoms are your digestive tract's way of sending signals of something that has gone wrong. Read these messages. Protect yourself against agonizing complaints. Make a few simple changes in eating methods. Use soothing foods for

[1]National Digestive Diseases Information Clearinghouse, 1986 survey, Washington, D.C. 20037

natural digestive aid. Pamper your tummy with these prudent corrective methods:

Eat but Do Not Overeat

Excessive food consumption slows down your stomach's normal activity. You have a sense of bloated fullness. Dyspeptic symptoms erupt when there is alteration of your stomach's normal motor activity. It is activated to churn comfortably when it is moderately distended with food. An overload means excessive stomach distention that blocks this churning activity to cause pains, bloating, and nausea. *Therapy:* Eat a balanced meal with moderate portions and not to the level of overstuffing. Something has to give, and it will be painful stomach symptoms!

Limit Fatty Food Intake

High-fat foods or those fried in fat inhibit stomach function and prolong the time before the stomach releases contents into the small intestine. An excess of fatty foods means double trouble with bloating due to overeating and also fat backlash with burning sensations. *Therapy:* reduce intake of animal fats. Avoid fried foods of any sort. Switch to vegetable fats, although also in moderation.

Avoid Tension While Eating

All tied up in knots? Feel anger, anxiety, resentment? This "uptight" frustration increases release of stomach acids to give you that "acid" indigestion. If a gas bubble carries some excess acid up into your esophagus or food tube, you suffer from heartburn. Feel depressed? This feeling of dejection reduces stomach acids and food remains undigested for many hours to give you cramps and common indigestion. *Therapy:* if emotionally upset, do *not* eat. A brisk 30-minute walk helps to calm your frazzled nerves. Drink a glass or two of comfortably cool water (*not* shocking cold or scalding hot!) and feel your tensions just wash away. Try one glass of skim milk about 1 hour before you eat. Its tryptophan (amino acid) releases serotonin (hormone) to ease your tensions and help you feel relaxed and ready to eat with comfort.

Eat Slowly for Your Stomach's Comfort

Eating rapidly or eating when emotionally upset is responsible for indigestion and uncomfortable spasms for hours afterward. If you have the "hurry up and eat" habit, you are abusing your digestive tract until it complains and begs you to slow down. *Therapy:* Use smaller utensils. Less food means less hurry. Chew well. Do not talk while you eat. Concentrate on the food and chewing it thoroughly for digestive comfort.

Do Not Swallow Air with Food

Air swallowing or *aerophagia* can lead to abdominal distention, smothering sensations, palpitations, and apparent heart pain. While some air is naturally swallowed with food and drink and nothing to worry about, large, disturbing amounts can give you distressing reactions. *Therapy:* Avoid gum chewing, smoking, drinking large amounts of carbonated beverages, engaging in animated mealtime conversations that lead to food gulping, and rapid eating. All bloat your system with pain-causing excessive air.

Some Foods May Not Like You

They may be nutritious, but for some folks, they cause indigestion and gasiness. Offenders include cucumbers, beans, cabbage, turnips, onions, chili, and peppers, to name a few. No matter how prepared or in minute amounts, they give you an unpleasant digestive reaction. *Therapy:* Keep a log of your foods. Do specific items cause digestive upsets? List these foods. Either reduce intake or eliminate them if you see they cause the problem. Often, just avoiding one offending food can help to correct the disorder.

HOW SIMPLE FIBER FOODS SOLVED A LIFETIME OF STOMACH TROUBLE—IN THREE DAYS!

Ever since he could remember, machine operator Stanley P. had recurring stomach pains. Either a grumble or a knifelike churning resulted in agony for hours on end. At times, he was doubled over with the stabbing pains and had to grit his jaw to keep from crying out. Antacids offered momentary relief, but when the effect wore off, the pains returned with greater vengeance. He worried that these pains, which began in his late teen years (and he was now approaching his forties), would plague him for the rest of his life.

A gastroenterologist asked about his diet pattern and noted a problem. Stanley P. ate almost no fiber or bulk-containing foods. The physician prescribed a daily intake of whole grain cereals for breakfast and chewy raw vegetables at lunch and dinner; he also told Stanley P. to include wheat germ and bran in his breakfast cereals, with any casseroles, or baked goods on a daily basis. Stanley P.

scoffed, expecting a patent medicine as a cure-all. But he was assured if it did not work, he would be given a prescription drug.

The machine operator used these fiber foods with his daily meals. Within *three days,* the painful spasms halted. He no longer felt shock waves shooting through his midsection after average foods. He was saved from a lifetime of digestive trouble by using small amounts of fiber foods on a daily basis. And they tasted good, too!

How Fiber Is a Form of Nutritional Therapy for the Digestive System

Lack of adequate amounts of fiber leaves you vulnerable to a gassy feeling that irritates your lower digestive tract. The painful spasm of excess gas occurs when your bowel wall becomes very sensitive to distention. Your goal is to protect against gas accumulation and speed up the release of waste products. You can do this with the use of high-fiber foods that hasten their expulsion. Fiber diminishes the amount of gas the body absorbs and makes for much smoother functioning along the gastrointestinal tract.

Nutritional Therapy

Boost intake of whole grain breads, cereals, raw fruits, and vegetables. Plan to have just one or two tablespoons daily of either bran or wheat germ (or a combo) to give you needed fiber to ease and erase stomach distress. Mix with cereals, into yogurt or in soups, stews, baked dishes for speedy correction of indigestion and its plaguelike symptoms.

How to Cool Off Scorching Heartburn

Problem: This disorder, more precisely called gastroesophageal reflux disease—or simply reflux, occurs when there is a backing up of stomach contents into the esophagus, the tube which connects the mouth to the stomach, causing a burning sensation commonly felt under the breastbone. Studies show that 67 million Americans experience heartburn at least once a month after eating a large meal or overindulging on certain foods. It can be both painful and alarming and is often understood. Almost 10 percent of patients who report to the hospital with severe chest pain are found to have no evidence of cardiovascular problems. Many, in fact, have reflux or heartburn.

126

While the most common symptom is the burning, there may also be regurgitation of bitter or sour fluid into the mouth. Other symptoms may include nausea, vomiting, bloating, and a persistent feeling of fullness after eating.

Are Medications the Solution?

Conventional antacids will neutralize the acid and relieve burning, but the physiology of the reflux remains uncorrected. Alginic acid combinations or "floating antacid foam" has no effect on delayed motility or weakened lower esophageal sphincter pressures. Anticholinergics impair gastric emptying and decrease lower esophageal sphincter (LES) pressure. H2 antagonists decrease acid secretion, but do not correct delayed emptying or improve LES tone. So you can see that you could be pouring oil on your flaming acid distress with most chemicalized medications. Hardly a soothing solution.

Instead, your goal is to correct the pathophysiology of reflux by (1) increasing LES pressure and (2) normalizing gastric emptying. In so doing, you improve the tone and amplitude of gastric contractions to facilitate normal emptying and reduce the amount of acidic contents available for reflux.

You can correct the cause and cool off that steaming cauldron of heartburn with this easy and speedily effective step-by-step nutritional and better living program:

1. Watch your weight. Lose that excess poundage. The pressure of extra weight can trigger more attacks of heartburn.

2. Avoid wearing clothing that is too tight around your stomach or waist.

3. Do not eat too fast. Take small mouthfuls and chew the food thoroughly.

4. Avoid bending forward, stooping, and lifting heavy objects.

5. Sleep with the head of your bed elevated about 6 inches (perhaps by placing wooden blocks or bricks under the legs at the head of your bed).

6. Keep a relaxed attitude in all your daily activities.

7. Do not lie down right after eating. And stop or cut down on your smoking.

8. Avoid any foods that may stimulate acid secretion in your stomach such as coffee, caffeine, alcohol, sugar, and salt.

9. Avoid fatty foods, as well as greasy, spicy foods. Cut down or eliminate chocolate.

10. Eat smaller, more frequent meals instead of the customary three large meals a day.

Nutritional Therapy

A cooling of heartburn is possible with a diet that is adequate in protein and low in fat. Enjoy broiled (or roasted) beef, poultry, and fish; also stock up on skim milk and related low-fat or fat-free dairy products. Soak up and cast out acid with potatoes, corn, apples, bananas, water, apple juice, soups (without garlic or onion, if offensive), and most freshly prepared raw fruits and vegetables.

Is Your Stomach Speaking to You?

If you eat any food that talks back in terms of heartburn, learn to avoid it. Or reduce its portion size. Your stomach is complaining. Better listen or pay the burning penalties afterward!

SIMPLE EVERYDAY MINERAL SUPPLEMENT PUTS OUT HEARTBURN FLAME IN TWO HOURS

Bertha K. felt recurring pains after any meal. The diagnosis of heartburn sent her on the merry-go-round of chemical medications that offered some relief but made her a habitual user of drugs. Without them, the flame reached right up to the roof of her mouth!

Fortunately, a nurse dietician at the school where Bertha K. taught told her she could find natural and nonaddictive relief from the use of a simple *calcium tablet!* She recommended a 500 milligram tablet with a glass of water after every meal to cool off the burning sensation. It would work within hours, assured the nurse.

Desperate, Bertha K. tried the calcium supplement after her dinner when she often felt the burning pain. She felt a slight warmth but it vanished and was comforted with a cooling sensation. It worked! She discarded her upsetting drugs and now takes just one 500 milligram calcium supplement after her dinner and has conquered the heartburn. And it went to work in dowsing the flame within two hours!

Why Calcium Is Effective Cooling Nutritional Therapy

Calcium imparts a mineral action that thickens stomach contents so they are less likely to move upward into the esophagus; it also helps to tighten comfortably and naturally the lower esophageal valve and protect against the upsurge of acid flow. Calcium may well be a natural treatment because it (1) strengthens lower esophageal sphincter, (2) stimulates stomach emptying to reduce chances of reflux, and (3) blocks acid from flowing back from the stomach into the esophagus. Just one 500 milligram calcium tablet, available at most health stores and pharmacies without prescription (it's in food!), can cool off your "hopeless" heartburn in a matter of hours or less!

How to Control a Hiatal Hernia

Problem: This is a condition in which part of the stomach slides up through the diaphragm (a thin muscle that separates the abdominal cavity from the chest cavity) into the chest area. While found in people of all ages, it is more common among those of the middle years. It is often painless. The symptoms—"heartburn," "indigestion," and various fright- ening pains—that bring people to the doctor's office are due to esophagitis, or irritation of the esophagus, which is very often but by no means always associated with hiatus hernia.

Checklist of Possible Causes

It may be an increase of pressure in the abdominal area produced by coughing, vomiting, straining the bowel or sudden physical exertion. Pregnancy, obesity or overweight, or the collection of fluid in the abdomen are also among the causes, since they all increase the pressure in the abdomen and tend to exert pressure on the stomach. If you correct the preceding causes, you may be relieved of the disorder.

Pressure, Stomach Acid, Irritation

Once a portion of the stomach protrudes through the diaphragm the effect is very much like what happens when you squeeze a toy balloon between your fingers: the pressure in the little protruding portion is increased. In hiatus hernia, the pressure inside the protruding portion of the stomach is increased to the point where it overpowers the valves that protect the esophagus from stomach acid. This acid becomes very irritating to the lining of the esophagus and produces some distress.

How to Gain Control and Overcome Hiatus Hernia

Nutritional Therapy

Make a checklist of which foods and drinks that cause distress. If highly spiced dishes irritate your esophagus, switch to better tolerated bland foods. Skim milk and whole grain crackers for a day or so should be soothing. Progress to whole grain cereals and pureed vegetables and some fat-free meats for a few weeks. Enjoy small and frequent feedings. Your last meal at night should be at least two hours before your go to bed. Avoid alcohol and carbonated beverages since they cause trouble to an inflamed esophagus. Of course, if you are overweight, there is another nutritional program in your future—a reducing diet.

The 5 Cent Food That Erases Hiatal Hernia

Just one tablespoon of ordinary bran is able to get to the root cause of your hiatal hernia and correct the errors that are to blame for your condition. That's right. All it costs is just 5 cents or less per day! For a lifetime of digestive super health!

Basic Cause

When you strain because of constipation or other difficulties, you raise tremendously the pressure in your abdominal cavity. This increased pressure causes the top of your stomach to push through your diaphragm to cause a hiatal hernia.

Nutritional Therapy

Ordinary bran, or "roughage," (which should be called "softage" because of its softening effect on hard wastes) is able to permit comfortable passage and *normalize* bowel functions. With the use of just 1 tablespoon daily of bran in your cereal or added to soups or stews or stirred in a cup of plain yogurt, you could help erase the risk of hiatal hernia almost at once. That's all it takes!

SAVED FROM SURGERY WITH BRAN AS HEALER

An examination of Edna E. showed that her hernia was in danger of becoming strangulated, that is, constructed in such a way as to cut off the blood supply. Her internist said that surgery might be necessary to reduce the hernia size and protect against strangulation. Was there an alternative? Obviously, Edna E. wanted to avoid surgery with its risks and doubts. Her internist said the condition was not yet that serious and the use of a pressure-relieving food could be tried. A patient exam told the doctor that Edna E. was constantly straining her bowel, which could be a clue to her developing condition.

Edna E. was told to add 1 or 2 tablespoons of bran daily to her diet. It would also consist more of whole grains, fresh fruits, and vegetables. This simple bran program worked! Eleven days later, a thorough exam indicated that she had corrected the condition and was spared surgery.

Why Bran Is a Lifesaver

Bran eases straining the bowel, permitting easier passage of waste and thereby cooling off any complicated esophagitis (inflammation); it also firms up the overworked lower esophageal sphincter. Introduce bran as part of your nutritional therapeutic program and protect against the distress of a hiatal hernia and other digestive disorders, too!

Nutritional Helps to Heal Your Ulcer

Problem: You know you may have a stomach ulcer when you feel a burning, gnawing pain, usually in the upper part of your abdomen, sometimes in your lower chest. It happens just after eating. The pain may endure for 30 minutes to 3 hours; it can come and go, with weeks of intermittent pain alternating with short pain-free periods. There are three basic types of ulcers that respond to nutritional therapy.

Duodenal Ulcer

An ulcer, or hole in the tissue, may be located in the part of the small intestine connected to the stomach. These duodenal ulcers are about four times more common than the other varieties.

Gastric Ulcer

This is an ulcer of the stomach lining or wall.

Peptic Ulcer

This ulcer occurs in either the duodenum (section of small intestine) or stomach of the digestive tract exposed to acid and pepsin (gastric juice).

Why Does It Happen?

The membrane lining the stomach and duodenum secretes a mucus that contains acid-neutralizing substances. This membrane protects the walls from being "eaten alive" by their own digestive juices. But if the lining cannot resist the damaging effects of acid and pepsin that are produced by the stomach to digest foods, the lining burns away and leaves the sore that is known as an ulcer.

Ulcers develop in older people who undergo a weakening of the stomach wall muscles, to the point where the muscles do not pound the food into liquid so readily. When solid food remains in the stomach for a long time, it stimulates excessive acid secretion which may cause gastritis—an inflammation of the stomach lining. Gastritis is considered to be a precursor of peptic ulcers.

A Nutritional Life-Style for Soothing and Healing Your Ulcer

A total stomach healing program calls for making adjustments in your life-style to give nutrition an opportunity to free you from ulcer distress. It's easy, effective, and quick, too!

1. *Forget the bland diet.* Being restricted to milk, pureed potatoes, and custards never did work. Instead, eat whatever you enjoy provided that the food or beverages make you feel good. Omit particular food that causes you discomfort. You *can* enjoy your favorite tangy foods if they are not irritating. Denying yourself enjoyable foods can worsen your condition because of the stress involved.

2. *Stress: Yes and no.* Stress *is* bad and any excess should be avoided, whether physical or emotional or a combination of both. The newer nutritional knowledge of ulcers holds that stress is *not* necessarily a

cause of ulcers, although it may contribute to the erosion. Many calm and relaxed persons develop ulcers; many high-stressed individuals are ulcer-free. There is no clear-cut cause-and-effect relationship between stress and ulcer onset.

3. *Give up smoking.* Smokers complain of stomach and duodenal ulcers twice as often as do nonsmokers; smokers are also more likely to have hemorrhage, perforation, and obstruction. Give it up! You may well give up your ulcer, too.

4. *Say "no" to aspirin.* It tends to cause internal bleeding and erosion of your stomach membranes; you already have that problem so why add to it? If you must take aspirin, ask your health practitioner if a child's product will do just as well (lower dosage) and wash it down with lots and lots of water.

5. *Limit or eliminate alcohol.* It may be involved in ulcer formation and certainly does aggravate an existing one. You would certainly never pour alcohol onto any open sore. Your ulcer is no exception.

Fit these life-style programs into your daily regimen, and you will help build resistance and hope for recovery from ulcer distress.

Seven Foods That Help to Heal Ulcer Sores

Vitamin A, via its predecessor of beta-carotene, is known for strengthening the epithelial cell layer (lining the stomach) and protecting against erosion from digestive juices. You can help nourish these eroded cells and sores and ulcerous wounds with an ample intake of those foods containing this "ulcer vitamin healer." Seven top-notch sources are sweet potatoes, carrots, pumpkins, winter squash, spinach, broccoli, and apricots. Include them in your weekly menu plan and you may well speed up the healing of ulcer sores!

Zinc

Zinc is able to protect against ulcers and speed up the healing of existing ulcers. Zinc blocks those chemical chain reactions that lead to ulcers by strengthening lysosomes (tiny sacs of enzymes in the cells of the stomach lining) and keeping them from spilling over into the membranes of the stomach. Zinc thereby acts as a barrier to shield your open sore from harmful substances. Food sources: Wheat germ, wheat bran, and cowpeas (blackeyes) are top-notch sources of this protective mineral.

Cabbage Juice

It has been reported that cabbage juice is helpful in easing and erasing the distress of an ulcer. An unidentified substance in the juice increases the resistance of the mucosal lining of the esophagus, stomach, and intestine to the erosive and ulcerating action of gastric juice, which is high in acid content and pepsin.

One Quart a Day May Keep Ulcer Away. In reported situations, 1 quart of cabbage juice a day was able to heal those who had ulcers at a much faster rate than on standard therapy. It was said that some patients healed after only 13 days with 1 quart of cabbage juice daily! Unavailable in packaged form, cabbage can be easily juiced or blenderized right at home.

Ice Water

Ice water has a shrinking effect on the stomach. It also decreases stomach acidity and will help to speed up healing of ulcers. Just one glass of ice water (especially a neutral pH mineral water) is much better than conventional milk, which stimulates acid secretion. If you drink up to five or six glasses of ice water throughout the day, you should find your ulcer easing up and perhaps ready to just "go away." (If you feel any discomfort from the ice water, sip slowly to adjust to the temperature.)

Barley

A bowl of barley, for breakfast or lunch or as a side dish at dinner, may be just what you need to help heal ulcers. It is a good source of thiamine, vitamin C, and calcium, all needed to repair the open sore. In particular, barley contains compounds that are said to neutralize acidity and ease the burning sensation. Barley is said to help repair the damaged DNA within the cells and accelerate the healing of the open sore.

When you eat barley, its natural mucilaginous content forms a protective barrier which keeps the acid juices away from the ulcer, allowing it to heal.

Any disturbance of the delicate balance between the aggressive forces of the digestive process and the defensive forces of the stomach is the forerunner of an ulcer. Nip this threat in the bud with the use of nutritional and better life-style therapies.

Is your stomach trying to tell you something? Listen to the protests. You may learn how to protect yourself from digestive disturbances and enjoy freedom from tummy distress!

HIGHLIGHTS

1. To cool off your raging stomach, follow the simple but effective corrective nutritional methods.
2. Stanley P. healed a lifetime of stomach trouble in three days with the use of fiber foods.
3. Cool off scorching heartburn with the 10-step improvement program.
4. Bertha K. turned to calcium tablets that extinguished heartburn flame in two hours.
5. Erase distress and threat of hiatal hernia with a simple 5 cent food.
6. Edna E. was saved from surgery with the use of bran for healing of her digestive problem.
7. A five-step program will help ease the distress of most ulcers.
8. Seven everyday foods have a vitamin that speeds up ulcer healing.
9. Cabbage juice promotes swift soothing healing of ulcer sores.
10. Cool off burning and acid irritating ulcers with ice water.
11. Daily use of barley will nourish your vital organs and repair ulcer and other sores.

Foods That Melt Body Fat, Control Appetite, and Keep You Slim and Trim

Clara H. wailed that all she had to do was look at food and she gained weight! She was embarrassed by her heavy midriff, thick thighs, bulging stomach. She knew she was the object of giggles when walking down the street. No matter what diet she tried, she seemed to gain back more than she lost!

Desperate, Clara H. brought her runaway appetite and heavy weight to a local diet specialist. She needed help for "the busiest jaws in town." The specialist explained that to control her compulsive eating, a few simple foods could correct the glandular malfunction that was the root cause of her voracious appetite.

Clara H. was given a set of foods that would create a simple but powerful hormonal reaction that would plug her eating urge. Desperate, Clara H. tried the foods either freshly prepared or as a juice. Within five days, she had lost 4 pounds. By the end of the month, she dropped two sizes. The greatest bonus was total self-control over her wild appetite. Within 60 days, she was a slimmer size eight...and still losing unwanted weight while her specialist noted she was healthier than ever. Now it was whistles instead of giggles that she heard when the slim-trim Clara H. walked down the street.

Fifteen Foods That Wash Excess Fat Out of Your Body

Clara H. was able to break up fatty deposits because certain foods actually counteract the cause of overweight by stimulating glands to release hormones to break up the fat-accumulating or *adipose* cells.

Why Fat Keeps Increasing

Adipose cells, when viewed through a microscope, appear as gray blobs enclosed in thin sheaths. The core of the cell—the *nucleus*—is also enclosed in a thin sheath. It is this core that serves as a storage depot for fat and causes a buildup of weight. When these cells accumulate too much weight, they begin to bulge. The fat becomes stored in the center of the cell, forcing the nucleus out to the cellular edge and locking the yellow fat in the core of the cell.

The body now has a tendency to develop more fat-storage cells which continually seek out fat. As more adipose cells develop, they become sluggish and cause the body's metabolic processes to slow down. This causes the body to become less efficient in burning up sugars and starches, thereby allowing carbohydrates to convert into stored-up fat. This leads to obesity and further development of fat-gathering cells.

Fat-Melting Foods

Your goal is to flush out the stored-up fat accumulated in your cells, and you can do this with the use of fat-melting foods as nutritional therapy. These foods have a natural diuretic action that unlocks and liquefies accumulated fats and washes them right out of your body. Slim your cells—and you slim your body.

Basic Program

Enjoy these foods (1) raw, (2) slightly steamed, or (3) as a juice. Plan to eat a variety throughout the week. If you eat or drink one or more *before* your meal, you will feel your appetite brought under control and you will be satisfied with smaller portions of food. You should have several of these fat-melting foods *every day,* for the cell-washing program to take hold and produce desired slimming results. Here is the set of important fat-melting foods that work from the first taste:

1. *Apples.* Apples are a prime source of pectin, enzymes, and vitamin C, which work to break down the hard blobs of fat in the cells to wash excess out of your system. Freshly chewed apples or apple juice will attack stored fat, uproot it, and prepare it for speedy elimination.

2. *Asparagus.* Slightly steamed, in a bit of oil, or blanched in water, asparagus is a prime source of an alkaloid known as asparagine. These alkaloids tend to stimulate the kidneys to break down fat and flush it out of your system.

3. *Beets.* Beets are a prime source of low-level iron, which cleanses fat cells and serves as a strong washing agent for flushing away

excessive deposits. Beets also contain natural chlorine, which helps scrub away fat that accumulates in the cells of your liver, kidney, and gallbladder. Chop up a raw beet in a salad and see your fat just vanish from your body.

4. *Cabbage.* The rich concentration of sulphur and iron serve as cleansing agents to wash out fat from your gastrointestinal area. Chopped raw, or slightly steamed cabbage or cabbage juice will perform the fat-washing result in moments.

5. *Carrots.* Carrots are a rich source of beta-carotene, the predecessor of vitamin A that accelerates your metabolism by nourishing your cells and triggering a fat-flushing reaction.

6. *Celery.* Fresh raw celery has a high concentration of calcium to energize your endocrine system, producing hormones that break down fatty buildup in the cells.

7. *Citrus fruits.* Try oranges, grapefruits, tangerines, lemons, and limes, which are rich in vitamin C and tend to reduce the effectiveness of fat. The vitamin liquefies and dilutes fat and then flushes it out of your body. Fruits also contain pectin, a natural fat-fighter that limits the amount of fat that adipose cells can absorb. When pectin substances are released in the system, they tend to absorb water and bombard adipose cells, thereby releasing clusters of fat.

8. *Cranberries.* Cranberries contain a natural enzyme that helps to break up fat accumulations and flush them out of your system. Cranberries are a vigorous natural diuretic with a high acidic content, needed to dislodge stubborn gluelike fatty deposits and eliminate them from your cells and body.

9. *Cucumber.* Cucumbers are a prime source of magnesium and alkaloids that work to disrupt fatty infestation and cleanse away the core of the sludge to slim your cells.

10. *Eggplant.* Unique amino acids are able to create glandular-hormonal reactions that vigorously scrub the fat from your cells and prepare for disposal through waste channels. Slightly steamed eggplant slices will offer good appetite control as well as fat-melting rewards in a short time.

11. *Oils, vegetable.* Vegetable oils are very beneficial in assisting in the breakdown and synthesis of accumulated fat in adipose cells. Once absorbed, just a tablespoon of oil acts as an insulator in maintaining body temperature. The essential fatty acids in the oils form impor-

tant constituents of cell membranes by regulating the intake and removal of wastes and transporting vital fat-insoluble nutrients.

12. *Parsley.* The potent vitamin A together with unique enzymes in *raw* parsley works wonders in prompting breakdown and removal of fatty deposits.

13. *Soybeans.* Cooked, of course, soybeans are a prime source of lecithin, which releases a by-product known as *lecithin cholesterol acyltransferase* (LCAT). This by-product serves as a barrier and defense mechanism for adipose cells. As fatty deposits are broken down with LCAT, they become more easily flushed from your system. A small portion of soybeans in a salad will act as natural appetite control and fat-fighter with the same bite! You eat, and reduce!

14. *Tomatoes.* Rich in vitamin C and natural citric acids, they assist in the speeding up of metabolic processes. Tomatoes and their juice act as a diuretic by stimulating the kidneys. This combination, with enzyme-activated minerals, signal your organs to filter fatty deposits from your bloodstream.

15. *Watermelon.* A unique fruit form of vitamin A and C together with the mineral-rich liquid join to break up fatty deposits and speedily wash them right out of your system.

Your Simple Fat-Washing Nutritional Therapy Program

Lose pounds and inches, firm up your unsightly flab, slim down in a short while by including a variety of these 15 fat-fighting foods in your daily program. *Example:* breakfast should include citrus and other fruits; lunch could include cucumber, eggplant, soybeans, and other vegetables; dinner could have just a variety of the vegetables. Just plan to eat *more* of these 15 foods throughout the days and weeks and watch that stubborn fat just wash right out of your body!

30 POUNDS JUST "VANISH" OVERNIGHT

Stuart I. kept letting out his belt until he had one notch left. His unsightly stomach spilled over his beltline. He had more than just "middle aged spread" (he was just 41), but was troubled with flabby thighs and heavy hanging buttocks and struggled to get up from his chair. He had tried various diet programs, but the fat clung to his midsection and elsewhere with stubborn determination. He wanted to get rid of the weight and appealed for help from a newly formed diet therapy program at the local medical facility.

Stuart I. was told to cut down intake of fatty meats and refined sugars. He argued he had tried this approach but with minimal and temporary success. The fat soon came back again. He was told by the medical specialists he needed to uproot and dislodge the fat that overwhelmed his adipose fatty tissue. He was to use the 15 fat-melting foods as part of his weekly menu. Less fatty foods and sugary sweets, but much, much more of these specific fat-fighters.

Stuart I. followed the program. Amazed, he could see his waistline shrinking day after day. His hips and thighs almost slenderized overnight, he would say. In no time at all, he had lost at least 30 fatty pounds. More weight was lost until he was slim with a 34-inch waistline and a lifeguard figure! With the use of the 15 fat-melting foods, he had conquered the fat problem by getting to the cause— overloaded cells. He was exhilarated because the program slimmed him so speedily or the pounds were able to "vanish overnight."

How Carbohydrate Foods Control Food Cravings

Facing a snack attack? Are you a compulsive eater? Can't control your appetite? Use food as a natural appetite suppressant to control these cravings. In particular, carbohydrates (fresh fruits, raw vegetables, and whole grains) create a biological reaction that puts a halt to your urge to overeat.

When you eat carbohydrates, your body releases a hormone, insulin, to process them. Insulin also influences the movement of tryptophan, an amino acid, to enter your brain to stimulate the release of serotonin. It is this "bathing" of your brain cells with serotonin that controls your urge to overeat. Serotonin is the substance that acts as an appetite suppressant. You are able to control runaway food cravings by this mechanism. Refer to Chart 11-1 for carbohydrate alternatives.

A Simple Orange Helps You to Avoid Overeating

A fresh orange that you eat slowly is a fast-acting food that "blocks" your urge to eat unnecessarily. It offers a quick-acting carbohydrate that raises your blood sugar and sends forth the brain-soothing serotonin that actually signals your senses to "turn off" your appetite.

Chart 11-1: CALORIE-CARBOHYDRATE CHART

A = average   C = cup   M = medium   Sm. = small   T = tablespoon
AS = average serving L = large   S = slice   Sq. = square   t = teaspoon

Item	Portion	Calories	Carbohydrate (grams)
Almonds	15	100	4
American Cheese	1S	100	Trace
Angel food cake	AS	200	32
Apple	M	50	22.6
Apple, dried, cooked without sugar	M	122	31.7
Apple juice	1 C	100	26
Apple dumpling	1 M	300	54
Apple pie	AS	350	51
Apple sauce	½ C	150	26
Apricots, dried	3 M	50	13.8
Apricots with syrup	3 M	75	26
Apricots	3 M	100	25
Apricot pie	AS	350	57.7
Asparagus soup	1 C	147	16.6
Bacon	1 S	30.5	.16
Banana	1 M	100	26
Banana split	A	400	92.5
Barley	¼ C	150	39
Bass	AS	100	0
Bean soup	1 C	170	22
Beans baked	½ C	261	47.77

Item	Portion	Calories	Carbohydrate (grams)
Beans, kidney	½ C	81	14.76
Beans, lima (baby)	½ C	94	17.84
Beans, string	1 C	44	10.2
Beef boiled	AS	250	0
Beef broth	1 C	30	3
Beef chopped	AS	100	0
Beef chuck/ground	AS	363	0
Beef/round steak	AS	292.32	0
Beets	¼ C	21	5
Berry pies	AS	350	56
Biscuits	1 Sm.	129	16
Blackberries	½ C	42.5	9.5
Blueberries	½ C	42.5	10.5
Bologna	2 S	150	2.2
Bouillon cube	1	2	0
Bran flakes	½ C	50	14
Bread, white	1 s	62	11.6
Broccoli	1 C	40	7
Brussels sprouts	⅔ C	36	6
Butter	1 Pat	50	Trace
Buttermilk	1 C	75	12

Chart 11-1: *(continued)*

Item	Portion	Calories	Carbohydrate (grams)
Cabbage boiled	¼ C	7	1.5
Cabbage, raw	¼ C	4	1
Candy, chocolate	1 oz.	133	17.8
Cantaloupe	½	115.5	28.87
Carrots	½ C	22.5	5
Catsup	1 T	25	4.2
Cauliflower	½ C	37	12.5
Celery	1 C	15	4
Cherries	1 C	133	33.06
Chicken, broiled	½ Sm.	281.52	0
Chicken, roasted	½ breast	106.08	0
Chicken soup	1 C	95	8
Chocolate cake	AS	205	29.12
Chocolate cookies	6 Sm.	108	17.16
Chocolate pudding	¼ C	80	62
Chocolate syrup	1 T	46.5	11.9
Cinnamon Toast	1 S	200	15.9
Clams	½ C	83	2.2
Cocoa with milk	1 C	212	27
Cocoa powdered	1 T	24.9	6.25
Codfish	AS	215	0

Item	Portion	Calories	Carbohydrate (grams)
Coffee, black	1 C	2.5	.66
Coffee cake	AS	90	14
Condensed milk	1 C	980	166
Consomme	1 C	21	1.92
Corn	¼ C	42.5	10
Corn flakes	½ C	50	11
Corn oil	1 T	125	0
Cottage cheese	1 T	21	.621
Crackers, soda	6	186	30
Cream	3 T	90	1
Cream cheese	1 oz.	104.72	.588
Cucumber	1 A	30	7
Cup cake	1 A	315	48
Doughnut	1 A	151	21.7
Duck	AS	109	0
Egg, hard-boiled	1	78	.4
Egg plant	½ C	19	4.1
Evaporated milk	1 C	345	.24

143

Chart 11-1: *(continued)*

Item	Portion	Calories	Carbohydrate (grams)
Filet of sole, broiled	AS	105.3	0
Flour, wheat	1 C	409	83.7
Frankfurter	1	182.4	.96
French dressing	1 T	100	3
Gelatin/sweetened	½ C	140	34
Grapefruit	½	50	13
Grapefruit juice	½ C	50	12
Grapes	1 C	65	15
Haddock, fried	AS	165	5.8
Halibut, broiled	AS	426	0
Ham	AS	126	0
Hamburger	2 oz.	363	0
Honey	1 T	65	17
Honeydew melon	¼	33	7.7
Ice cream	1 C	290	29
Jam	1 T	55	14
Kale	½ C	28	4.86
Lamb chop	1 M	260	0
Lamb roast	AS	119	0
Lemon	1 M	20	10.7
Lemon pie	AS	305	45
Lentils	½ C	233	41.7

Item	Portion	Calories	Carbohydrate (grams)
Lettuce	¼ Head	15	3
Liver, calf	AS	74	1.7
Lobster, broiled	1	308	.8
Macaroni	1 C	190	39
Mackerel, broiled	AS	415.2	0
Meat loaf	AS	264	11.5
Milk, skim	1 C	90	12
Milk, whole	1 C	161	12
Muffins	1	125	17
Mushrooms	⅔ C	26.6	4
Mustard	1 T	3.5	.32
Nectarine	1 M	80	21.37
Noodles	½ C	100	18
Oatmeal	½ C	65	16
Okra	½ C	34.2	7.92
Olive oil	1 T	125	0
Olives	3 Sm.	15	Trace
Onion raw	1 M	40	10
Onion cooked	3 M	180	42
Orange	1 M	75	14
Orange juice	1 C	110	26
Oysters, raw	12	104	5

Chart 11-1: CALORIE-CARBOHYDRATE CHART (continued)

Item	Portion	Calories	Carbohydrate (grams)
Parmesan cheese	1 T	25	Trace
Parsnips	1 M	121	28
Peaches canned	1 C	200	52
Peaches fresh	1 M	35	10
Peach pie	AS	421	63
Peanut butter	1 T	93	3.12
Peanuts	¼ C	336	11.16
Pears, fresh	1 Sm.	100	25
Pears, canned	1 C	195	50
Pears, dried	½	50	13
Peas	¼ C	21.2	3.9
Pecans	1 C	740	16
Peppers, green	1 M	15	4
Pimento cheese	1½ oz.	150	2.8
Pineapple, fresh	1 S	37.44	9.86
Pineapple, canned	1 S	45	12
Pineapple, pie	AS	404	61
Plums, canned	1 C	205	53
Plums, fresh	1	25	7
Powdered sugar	1 T	30	8
Pork chop broiled	1 M	101.6	0
Pork roast	AS	380.1	0
Pork sausage	2	188	0

Item	Portion	Calories	Carbohydrate (grams)
Postum, no milk	1 C	10	2
Pot roast	AS	339.3	0
Potato, baked	1 Sm.	141	32
Potato, boiled	1 M	110.2	24.79
Potato chips	1 chip	11	1.0
Potato, french fried	10 pieces	155	20
Potato mashed	½ C	62.5	12.5
Potato salad	½ C	99	16.3
Potato soup	1 C	105	12
Potato sweet	1 M	15	4
Prunes	3	52.5	13.5
Prune juice	½ C	100	24
Pumpkin pie	AS	275	32
Radishes	5 M	10	1.8
Raisin pie	AS	325	32.5
Raisins	¼ C	125	128
Raspberries, canned	½ C	50	21.4
Raspberries, fresh	½ C	50	23.5
Rhubarb, stewed	1 C	211	54
Roast beef	AS	261	0
Roquefort cheese	AS	150	.5
Roquefort dressing	1 T	125	1.2

Chart 11-1: CALORIE-CARBOHYDRATE CHART (continued)

Item	Portion	Calories	Carbohydrate (grams)
Round steak	AS	254	0
Rutabaga	½ C	35	8.2
Ry-Krisp	5	100	19.2
Salmon, red	1 C	427	0
Sardines	3	233	.45
Sauerkraut	½ C	27.5	4.5
Scallops, steamed	1 C	112	0
Shrimp, breaded	1	31.97	4.57
Sirloin steak	AS	261	0
Sour cream	1 T	30.3	.625
Spaghetti	1 C	155	32
Spinach	½ C	20	3
Squash, hubbard	½ C	36	8.9
Squash, summer	¼ C	15	3.5
Strawberries	1 C	55	13
Succotash, canned	½ C	89	19.7
Sugar white	1 t	20	6
Swiss cheese	1 S	68	Trace

Item	Portion	Calories	Carbohydrate (grams)
Tangerine	1 L	40	10
Tapioca pudding	½ C	100	11.6
Tea plain	1 C	2	.4
Tomato	1	40	9
Tuna, cooked	1 C	315	0
Turkey	AS	70.4	0
Turnips	½ C	18	4
Veal chop	1 M	107.6	0
Vegetable soup	1 C	84	9
Watercress	1 C	4	.6
Watermelon	1 S Sm.	115	27
Wheaties	½ C	75	12
Whipped cream	3 T	30	Trace
White fish steamed	AS	275.8	0
Yams	1 M	210	48.2

Try Quick-Acting Appetite Tamers

Quiet those food grumblings by eating just one or two of these complex carbohydrate foods: oranges, grapefruits, apples, pears, peaches, plums, watermelons, bananas, figs, nectarines, pineapples, tangerines, or pitted prunes.

Eat Slowly to Improve Brain Signals

Peel and/or wash the fruit. Chew slowly. The gradual mastication and swallowing will maximize the release of tryptophan and serotonin, which influence the neurotransmitters in your brain to "turn off" the runaway urge to eat. Within a few minutes, you will have soothed your compulsive desire to snack and gained control over your own willpower. It is this brain chemistry of nutritional therapy that controls your craving for high-calorie foods.

Two Weight-Control Tonics That Work
in Minutes

To ease your desire to eat excessively, try these weight-control tonics that work swiftly to tame your taste buds and give you a comfortable feeling, even though you have not eaten a thing.

Ice Water Plus Lemon Twist

Many restaurants serve you ice water before a meal so you will be satisfied with smaller portions. Try this same trick to control your weight. Ice water, with a bit of lemon twist flavor, will "shrink" your stomach muscles and give you that satisfied fullness to ease and eliminate eating urges. Try it whenever you have a snack attack!

Vegetable Juice + Garlic Clove = Hunger Satisfaction

A glass of salt-free vegetable juice together with a mashed or diced garlic clove works wonders in soothing your appetite and giving you speedy hunger satisfaction. The complex carbohydrates of the vegetable juice are stimulated by the garlic's *gastroenteric allichalon* to give you a sedative action by delaying excessive motor activity of your stomach. In moments, your hunger pangs are eased. The grumblings are ended. Your eating urges are under control. *Tip:* Begin your meal with this vegetable juice plus garlic combo, and you will be satisfied with much smaller portions.

With either or both of these weight-control tonics, you help put a "hold" on your appetite and also set off a chain reaction to wash out the fat from your cells and bring down your waistline and other bulges.

CONTROL NERVOUS APPETITE, LOSE WEIGHT IN SEVEN WEEKS

Marge N., a publicist for a large entertainment facility, was always edgy. Instinctively, she would munch and nibble and eat more than she should. Her weight ballooned until she had a matronly look in a profession that demanded sleek and youthful slimness at any age.

She experienced side effects from chemical appetite suppressants that were threatening to become addictive. She asked a backstage nurse in attendance if there were any alternatives to these drugs. She was told to alternate between the ice water–lemon twist tonic and the vegetable juice–garlic clove tonic. Marge N. tried both. Immediately, her appetite calmed and her weight started to go down along with reduced food consumption. In seven weeks, she was sleek and trim again and joked she could appear in a commercial as the "after" half of a successful weight loss program. And all it took were the natural weight-control tonics!

It's Time for Your Personal Size-Up!

Instructions

Tape together some large sheets of construction paper the length of your height and spread the paper on the floor. Lay on top of it. Have a friend draw an outline of your body, starting with feet on up to your head. Now pin the paper to the wall and give it a long, hard look.

Scenario

Not exactly happy with what you see? Think you'd like to erase about 10 to 15 pounds of bulging lines from the picture? You may want to lose for an upcoming special event—graduation, a wedding, or a party. Whatever the reason, you want to look your best and bring out the beauty that's in you. The problem is, you don't want an unsafe crash diet or to spend months trying to lose. But a fast-weight-loss diet that's also well-balanced nutritionally can be coupled with a regular program of exercise, to bring your shape "in line."

Habits, nasty habits Why did you let yourself get out of shape? Somewhere along the line your behavior got out of hand. You have old habits about eating and thinking "fat," so whenever you start dieting you have myriad excuses: "It's impolite to turn food down"; "My mother forced me to clean my plate"; and "My job is demanding and I need something to relieve the tension." Whatever your excuses are for poor eating habits, you'll find a way to reinforce them. But let's face it, you'll eat for the rest of your life, so sacrificing a few mouthfuls here and there to be trim isn't going to hurt. It's time to control your life, not let food control you.

The following quiz is designed to reveal your savviness—or lack of it—in the areas of diet and exercise. The perfect score is 100; answering 75 percent of the questions means you're ahead of the game; anything below 50 means you've got a lot of work to do.

Questions

	True	False
1. A few extra calories a day won't make a difference in my weight.	☐	☐
2. Exercising will make me hungry, I'll eat more and never lose weight.	☐	☐
3. In order to see any results in fitness I have to exercise vigorously every day.	☐	☐
4. Calisthenics are more gentle and better for my health than aerobics.	☐	☐
5. A banana has less calories than a yogurt bar.	☐	☐
6. The body needs more protein than carbohydrates.	☐	☐
7. Ice cream is more fattening than frozen yogurt.	☐	☐
8. Once water weight is eliminated, you start losing fat on a starvation diet.	☐	☐
9. Playing tennis (singles) is more active than bicycling vigorously.	☐	☐
10. Red meats have more calories than fish or poultry because they're higher in fat.	☐	☐

Answers

1. *False.* Eating 100 extra calories a day can add 10 pounds a year to that svelte body of yours.

2. *False.* People who spend a great deal of energy on vigorous exercise may need extra calories. But regular, moderate exercise *doesn't* increase the appetite and may actually reduce hunger.

3. *False.* After rigorous exercise muscles need 48 hours to recover from the minor damage they may incur from the workout. Most exercise training programs suggest you work-out every other day to avoid this injury.

4. *False.* While stretching exercises are beneficial in toning the body and increasing flexibility, aerobics is the best all-around exercise for your body. Include swimming, jumping, running, or walking—a continuous workout for 15–30 minutes, three to four times a week, on alternate days. Aerobics helps strengthen the heart, lung, and circulatory systems and helps to *manage weight.*

5. *True.* A banana, nature's portable snack food, not only has fewer calories (about 100) than a yogurt bar (125 calories), but is high in potassium, low in sodium, almost fat-free, and provides vitamins A and C.

6. *False.* The body needs less protein than carbohydrates! Fruits and vegetables, whole grains and pastas, should make up 55 percent of the diet; fat 30 percent; and finally, protein, 12–20 percent.

7. *True.* Ice cream may have more calories, but, fruit-flavored frozen yogurt should not be considered "low in calories" because of its high sugar content. Read the labels on ice cream and yogurt carefully for fat and sugar contents—and calories.

8. *False.* You actually start losing lean tissue and not fat—so your body tries to replace the muscle tissue, encouraging weight to bounce back.

9. *False.* Tennis burns 450 calories per hour, while bicycling at 10 m.p.h. burns up 510 calories.

10. *True.* Broiled halibut, 3½ oz. has 171 calories; the same amount of roast chicken, white meat, has only 166 calories; a broiled, untrimmed sirloin steak, however, has *387* calories.

How Exercise Unlocks the Bottled-up Body Fat for Swift Melting

Food therapy plus exercise will get rid of accumulated body fat. This combination is the key to successful weight loss. Simply speaking, in 1 pound of body fat, there are about 3,500 calories. If you eat 3,500 more calories than your body needs, it stores up that pound. But if you eliminate 3,500 calories, you lose a pound. Controlled nutrition is one-half of the fat-washing process. Simple exercise is the second half of the picture. (See Chart 11-2, which lists various activities and the calories they burn.)

Chart 11-2: 100 CALORIE ACTIVITY CHART

To burn up 100 calories, you must

Walk (briskly)	16 minutes
Climb stairs	5 minutes
Iron clothes	24 minutes
Make beds	19 minutes
Scrub floors	17 minutes
Shovel snow	14 minutes
Play basketball	12 minutes*
Play Ping-Pong	21 minutes
Swim	8 minutes
Play golf	18 minutes
Play tennis	14 minutes
Bowl	12 minutes*
Row	13 minutes
Dance	25 minutes
Horseback-ride	33 minutes
Bicycle	13 minutes
Jog	8 minutes
Ski (downhill)	9 minutes
Ski (cross-country)	5 minutes

*Of active playing time.

During exercise, your body speeds up its basal metabolism rate and activity level. At the same time, it alerts a weight-regulating center (your hypothalamus or a pea-sized segment of your brain) that balances energy use with food consumption.

Just as you have internal controls to keep your body temperature constant, you also have a thermostat for fat. You need to raise that thermostat to help burn up the accumulated fat in your cells. This activity causes enzymatic changes that accelerate fat metabolism in your tissues.

Simple Walking Is Effective

If you walk 1 hour a day for 10 days, you will burn up about 350 calories each day or 3,500 calories at the end. You will have lost 1 pound of fat. It is a simple but effective way of helping to control caloric-fat buildup.

How Exercise Controls Your Appetite

Contrary to popular belief, exercise does *not* increase your appetite. It has a reverse benefit. It *depresses* your appetite. In brief, since blood sugar is the primary source of energy for the brain, a *low blood sugar level* can make you feel hungry. However, when you exercise, fat is released into your bloodstream to be utilized as a fuel to produce energy instead of the body using blood sugar. This enables your blood sugar to remain relatively constant, and therefore you will not feel hungry since your body is *burning fat* rather than utilizing sugar as its source of energy.

The biological changes that occur during and immediately following exercise are especially important since you will want to do an exercise about 1 hour before mealtime. Subsequently, you will experience a *decrease in your appetite.*

Plan to do 30 to 60 minutes of exercise 1 hour before you eat and then another 30 to 60 minutes 1 hour after you eat. This simple program will help wash away fatty overload and keep your cells slim and trim.

Foods That Work as Natural Fat Busters

To lose weight rapidly, a key factor is in activation of physiological processes to uproot the stored fat. You do this by stimulating your sympathetic nervous system to pour forth a substance called norepinephrine. This substance is then able to accelerate a metabolic process that zeroes in on your fat cells to help dislodge and disperse the globules to be washed out of your system.

Foods That Increase Fat-Busting Action

To wake up your nervous system and induce a flow of fat-washing norepinephrine, you need to eat small portions of those foods containing tyramine, an amino acid. It is tyramine that triggers the release of norepinephrine, the key to fat busting.

Food Sources of Tyramine: Consider the avocado, pineapple, banana, plum, lemon, tangerine, tomato, potato, eggplant, and apple cider vinegar. *Cheeses include* Brie, Roquefort, Edam, Gruyère, Limburger, brick, American, Swiss, Camembert, bleu, cheddar, Gouda, Munster.

How to Use Food As Fat Busters. Eat a small portion of any of these foods with your meal. All you need, for example, would be a slice or two of pineapple, or one banana, or one tomato in your salad with a sprinkle of apple cider vinegar and lemon, or else a small square of cheese, about 1 or 2 tablespoons, with an apple for dessert. Almost at once, the tyramine will initiate an outpouring of norepinephrine to work as fat busters to slim your cells. A little bit will go a long way.

Caution: Some groups of people should be careful about foods containing tyramine. If you have a history of migraine headaches, this amino acid could be upsetting. Or if you are taking prescribed monoamine oxidase inhibitors (antidepressants and blood pressure drugs), you should check with your health practitioner before increasing your intake of tyramine.

With the use of these nutritional therapies, you will be able to control your appetite and ease the hunger urge, soothe stomach pangs, and help lose unsightly and unhealthy weight in a short time.

Fight Fat with Behavior Control

You may eat sensibly all week, but if you help yourself to extra servings of cakes on the weekends, extra pounds will start to bulge. Most people become less active as they grow older, and this has the same result as eating more. With additional pounds to carry around, you become less active, add more fat, and so on in a vicious spiral interrupted only by periodic stints of dieting.

Maintaining a sensible weight does not mean a lifetime of carrots and celery, nor does it require hours of grueling calisthenics, but it does mean keeping calorie consumption and activity in harmony. It's like balancing a checkbook, and the human body is a strict account! Change your behavior, make a commitment, establish new patterns, and you will get rid of your pounds and keep pounds from coming back.

Make Simple Adjustments for Fast Weight Loss

Try taking smaller portions of food at meals. Still hungry? If you go back for seconds, you will be eating because you want the food, not just because it is on your plate. *Tip:* Put foods out of sight. Don't leave candies, nuts, crackers, or goodies around the house. If you find you listen to the clock rather than your stomach, go without a watch, or rearrange your schedule so when it is time to eat, you are busy with something else.

Be a Slower Eater

If you are one of the faster forks around, slow down. Put your fork down between bites. Chew each mouthful thoroughly. *Reason:* fast eating doesn't give your body a chance to react to the food you've eaten. By the time your body is able to say, "that's enough," you've already had too much. *Solution:* eat what seems a reasonable amount and leave the table for 30 minutes. Still hungry after half an hour, then go back to the table and resume your meal. You may well find you no longer feel so hungry, if at all.

If you wail that everything you look at or touch turns to fat, then dry your tears and start using nutritional therapies that let you eat and control your appetite while you lose unwanted weight in a jiffy.

BEST POINTS

1. Clara H. used an assortment of fat-washing foods that controlled her eating urges, soothed her appetite, and made her slim and trim in a short time.
2. Use any of the tasty 15 fat-washing foods and beverages as nutritional therapies to control your weight the easy way.
3. Stuart I. saw 30 pounds just "vanish overnight" on a simple fat-washing program with the 15 foods.

4. Everyday carbohydrate foods can control your eating urges by acting on the appetite center of your brain.

5. Two immediately prepared weight-control tonics use all-natural ingredients to help strengthen willpower and "turn off" your eating urges.

6. Marge N. controlled her nervous appetite and lost excess weight in seven days with the use of two tonics using everyday ingredients.

7. Use the self-test, the calorie-carbohydrate chart, and the fitness guide to help speed up your weight-loss program.

8. Enjoy the tyramine-containing foods that speed up fat busting.

9. A few simple behavior adjustments will ease fast weight loss.

12

How to Use Nutritional Therapy as Pain Relievers

"Take two aspirin and call me in the morning," is the familiar prescription for most common aches and pains. While medication will ease the pain, when the effect wears off, the distress returns again and again. Constant hurt, whether a headache, low-back pain, arthritis, or neuralgia, is a vicious circle which leads to irritability and depression. In many situations, the victim cannot sleep at night. Next day's weariness compounds the problem, leading to more nervousness and pain. In desperation, reaching for a medicated pain killer seems to be the only solution.

Are Medications the Answer to Pain?

Whether it is acetaminophen, aspirin, ibuprofen, or any of the other extrastrength, double-power medications that promise swift (although temporary) relief for the pain, there are penalties. These analgesics (pain relievers) lead to side effects such as acute liver damage, nausea and vomiting, ringing in the ears, sweating, flushing, fever, hyperventilation, slurred speech, gastric irritation, drowsiness, internal bleeding. You may ease the pain, but you are exchanging one disorder for another, which could be more serious! Clearly, medications are not the solution to pain.

Why Does It Hurt?

One reason is that nerve endings sensitive to touch are pressed very hard. Neuroscientists have found that your body is covered with many small nerve cells with extremely fine nerve fibers that are excited exclusively by intense, potentially harmful stimulation. Scientists call the nerve cells *nociceptors,* from the word noxious, meaning physically harmful or destructive. It's as if nature has sprinkled your body with a variety of pain-sensitive cells, not only to report what kind of hurt you're experiencing, but to make sure the message gets through. They reach your central nervous system and send forth agonizing signals.

How Your Body Can Be Taught to Block Pain

You can control and block the spread of pain when you consider a pain-suppressing pathway involving the "gate theory." That is, when pain signals first reach the nervous system, they excite a group of neurons until a hypothetical "gate" opens up to allow pain signals to be sent to higher brain centers. But the good news is that nearby neurons in contact with the pain cells can suppress activity so that the gate stays closed. It calls for the use of certain nutrients that strengthen the cells to release vital pain-suppressing substances called *endorphins.* In effect, the body "closes the gate" to block pain. These endorphins promote the flow of a soothing balm to quiet nerve cells, block and ease, and even erase pain. To help your body produce these morphinelike (but all-natural) pain killers, specific nutrients are needed in small, but quickly effective, amounts. These nutrients can block pain!

The Protein That Is an All-Natural Pain Killer: Phenylalanine

A nutritional amino acid, found in everyday foods, and available as a food supplement, holds the key to ending chronic pain. This all-natural pain killer, *phenylalanine,* is an essential amino acid that your body cannot make but must be obtained from foods or a supplement.

Phenylalanine works by protecting endorphins, your pain-relieving substances that move through your nervous system to make you feel relieved in body and mind. (This amino acid also lifts depression and brightens your blue moods.) The nutrient energizes the activity of your endorphins to help make you immune to pain, speaking broadly.

Phenylalanine Power for Swift Pain Relief

As an example, we have beta-endorphin which is said to be 50 times stronger than morphine, the strongest chemical pain killer we have. Yet, it is phenylalanine that protects beta-endorphin from natural destruction so it can act as an all-natural pain reliever for what ails you.

How to Use Phenylalanine

This isolated amino acid is available as a supplement. Swift pain relief has been noted for those who follow this simple program: 375 milligrams with breakfast, 375 with lunch, and another 375 with dinner. It is effective if taken *with* your meal or within 5 minutes after finishing your meal.

Almost immediately, the amino acid boosts the production of endorphins to help "close the gate" of pain by pouring forth the soothing balm to calm nerve cells. Before the day is over, your pain should have vanished.

Food Sources of Phenylalanine

Stock up on nonfat milk, cheddar cheese, turkey, rolled oats, shredded wheat, peas, corn, and lima beans. Calves' liver is a potent source but also extremely high in cholesterol and fat so you trade off one benefit for another blood fat risk. *Suggestion:* include moderate portions of nonfat milk and the other foods in your weekly eating guide to help protect your supply of endorphins and keep the "gate" closed to banish pain. But you would have to consume a large amount of such foods to act as "natural pain killers" so it makes good sense to use a supplement in the suggested potencies for swift relief, the easy way.

FREED FROM LIFETIME OF HEADACHES WITH NUTRIENT

For many years, Jim R. suffered the excruciating pain of cluster headaches. Night after night, throughout the day, the pain kept throbbing without relief. He was nervous, irritable. He was only 48 years old, when the stubborn pain threatened his job as a systems analyst. His entire livelihood in jeopardy, he sought help from a nutritionally oriented medical staff at a nearby pain clinic. He was told to take the nutrient, phenylalanine, in potencies just as described (375 milligrams). He was directed to halt temporarily taking prescribed medications that gave him agonizing side effects with minimal relief. Results? In four days, his formerly "hopeless" headaches ended. By taking the phenylalanine just one day per week, in the three suggested dosages, he has become free of the pains, and the medicines, too!

Foods That Soothe Muscle Pains

Do you wince with spasms when you have to move your shoulder? Troubled with a shooting pain in your hips when you try to stand up or get out of bed in the morning? Are you troubled by stiff and painful neck and back muscles and joints?

To answer the pain alarm, you may be taking prescribed or over-the-counter patent remedies. There is some temporary relief, but when the effect wears off, the agony returns with even more ferocious attack. The reason is that you need to get to the *root cause* of your muscle pain. Namely, your protective endorphins need to be gathered and activated from your brain nerve cells to inhibit movement of pain-causing cells into your muscles and joints.

Magnesium Is Most Soothing

This mineral is able to boost production of the protective endorphins to inhibit the dispersion of the pain-causing cells that threaten your muscles and joints. Magnesium is a valuable part of bone and soft tissue and is needed to maintain stability of your nerves and muscles. A deficiency of magnesium can cause hyperirritability of nerves and muscles, tissue weakness, irregular heartbeat, and eventually spasms and convulsions. It is magnesium in foods that will not only soothe muscle pains, but *prevent* them.

Food Sources of Magnesium

These include brewer's yeast, wheat bran, wheat germ, green leafy vegetables such as kale and beet greens, nuts, brown rice, and soybeans.

Untie Muscle Spasms with Magnesium

The gnarled tight feeling in your muscles and joints could be a signal that your body needs magnesium to untie those agonizing knots. With this mineral, your enzyme system becomes activated, and there is an improved fat and electrolyte metabolism to improve your muscular flexibility. In moments, your "knots" are untied, and you have greater mobility of your muscles and joints. More important, you are free of the stubborn pain.

How to Take Magnesium as a Pain Killer

For a margin of safety, women should have at least 400 milligrams per day, and men should take close to 700 milligrams per day. This plan will meet needs even under increased requirements such as heavy stress.

You may also be magnesium nourished by ingesting the foods listed as being rich in this pain-killing mineral. For example, consider this tonic:

Magnesium Tonic. Blenderize green leafy vegetables together with 1 teaspoon brewer's yeast, 1 teaspoon wheat bran, 1 teaspoon nuts. Just one 8-ounce glass will give you a powerhouse of magnesium along with other vitamins and minerals to provide swift relief for your muscle pain. Best of all, it has a refreshing taste and is all natural! A glass of Magnesium Tonic a day will keep your muscle pain away!

FREES HERSELF FROM NECK PAIN IN ONE HOUR

An avid reader, Peggy MacD., was constantly troubled with neck and back pain. Working days at a video display terminal and reading hours at night, took their toll. Her tensed head and neck muscles felt as if they were being squeezed between two giant hands.

Peggy MacD. was an "aspirin addict" in a desperate effort to ease the pain. Postural changes offered only minimal help. When she experienced dizziness and nausea from the medication, she felt helpless. She visited the company physician who noted her blood levels of magnesium were very low. He suggested a magnesium supplement in doses of just 500 milligrams per day for just a week. Then she was to take the Magnesium Tonic as a means of boosting her supply of this muscle-soothing mineral.

Peggy MacD. took the supplement. Within 1 hour, the pain was gone! She took magnesium for the recommended week. Then she took the refreshing tonic. The pain never returned! Now she could read and work and be free of the viselike tortuous neck–back muscle contractions, thanks to the miracle mineral of magnesium!

The Simple Grain That Soothes Morning Stiffness

Just include 1 tablespoon of wheat bran with your morning breakfast cereal. Stir it in to mix with the other grains. You have a powerhouse of concentrated magnesium that works wonders right in the morning to unlock your aching muscles and take the kinks out of your joints so you have youthful flexibility the day ahead!

Suggestion: For more vigorous and speedy action, add an additional ½ teaspoon of brewer's yeast and ½ teaspoon of wheat germ to your breakfast cereal, along with the wheat bran. You now have a triple-power in fighting and eliminating joint-muscle pain in the morning so you can face the day ahead with a cheerful mind and body. (They do go together!)

Calcium Can Cool That Burning Pain

When agonizing pain strikes, it is often accompanied with a burning or inflammation that can best be described as somewhat feverish. The area is not only subjected to stabbing aches but heat spasms that intensify when you try to move the area. Anti-inflammatory drugs are available to provide temporary relief, but they also carry the risk of side effects. Furthermore, when the drugs wear off, there is a return of the pain and the inflammation that always seems worse than before. Is there a nutritional therapy as alternative? Yes, it is in the form of calcium.

How Calcium Eases Overheated Pain

Calcium plays a vital role in maintaining the natural muscle and nerve reaction to function without distress. Calcium guards against painful twitching or spasms of the muscles. This mineral is required for normal nerve transmission to help ease muscular stress and keep the area feeling cool and relaxed.

Stress, Pain, Calcium

Chronic, unrelieved emotional and/or physical stress opens the "gate" to permit outpouring of pain. Unrelieved stress causes stiffness to build up as nerve reflexes reduce circulation, leading to increased pain. Messages sent over nerve pathways bring on inflammation and distress. Because the neck and the rest of the back are so closely related structurally, if you have a problem in one area, you may eventually have problems in the other area. And it can all be worsened with stress.

Calcium is a mineral that is able to soothe nerves to protect against irritability; this mineral is responsible for the alternate contraction and relaxation of body muscles. You know calcium soothes your stressful aches when you drink a glass of warm milk and feel yourself relaxing all over. You can use calcium to cool off your burning pain and protect against return of these distressful symptoms.

How to Use Calcium to Heal Pain

The simplest and swiftest pain reliever would be a glass of warm milk (low-fat, if possible). You could boost the calcium content by stirring in 2 or 3 tablespoons of nonfat dry milk powder into the fluid milk. Within moments, the calcium is stabilizing the spasms, soothing your stress, releasing the endorphins needed to block pain signals. You heave a sigh of relief, thanks to calcium as a pain reliever.

Other Stress-Soothing, Pain-Easing Calcium Sources

One ounce of Gruyere cheese or cheddar cheese or soybean tofu, will give you a rich concentration of calcium needed to make you feel soothed and relaxed all over. You could also try ½ cup of canned salmon, bones and all, for quick relief of aching stiffness.

HOW SIMPLE SNACKS HELP TO AVOID PAIN ATTACKS

Because Benjamin X. had a stressful position as sales supervisor, having to deal with personality clashes, he was given to frequent attacks of stiff neck, low-back pain, arthritic like gnarled shoulder muscles. Medications gave little help, but many side effects. He had frequent pain attacks that lasted for the whole day. A few days of relief, then the attacks struck again, sometimes longer, sometimes shorter. He asked help from a company dietician and was told to "snack" on calcium foods. He carried a small thermal container with chunks of the high-calcium cheeses. For lunch, he would have a salmon salad with a scoop of low-fat cottage cheese (more calcium). On occasion, he would have a glass of warm skim milk in the company cafeteria. Within four days, this simple snack program gave Benjamin X. total freedom from pain attacks. As long as he had a small chunk of cheese each day, he was able to enjoy immunity against the debilitating pain that had so plagued his working days and nights, too. Calcium had soothed his stress and eased and even erased his pain.

The Protein That Protects You Against Pain: Tryptophan

Tryptophan is more than a building block of protein. It is one of the most potent (and natural) pain relievers available. It has been called the best and safest nondrug remedy for most pain. Yet, it is scarce in the typical American diet, suggesting a possible reason for the widespread prevalence of pain.

How Tryptophan Blocks Pain

This amino acid is a predecessor of serotonin, a neurotransmitter in the brain, which energizes the activity of endorphins, your body's own

163

pain killers. Your pain perception threshold comes under your control with the availability of this protein.

Tryptophan also induces a desire for relaxation as well as sleep. You will not fall into a deep sleep when having a tryptophan supplement, but you will be totally relaxed and calmed down in body and mind when the serotonin bathes your nerve cells and tissues and unties the knots in your muscles.

How to Take Tryptophan

For best results, take it between meals with a low-protein food such as fruit juice or whole grain bread (otherwise, other amino acids in a high-protein meal tend to crowd tryptophan out and prevent it from reaching your brain).

Plan to eat a high-carbohydrate, low-fat, and low-protein meal, even though protein is the only dietary source of tryptophan. *Reason:* When protein is digested, tryptophan enters the bloodstream and joins a pool of other amino acids waiting to be transported to your brain. But the carrier molecule designed to do that also carries eight other amino acids. The object is to tip the balance in favor of tryptophan.

That is where the high-carbohydrate diet plan comes into the nutritional therapy picture. After eating a meal high in carbohydrates, the body releases insulin. And this hormone in turn facilitates the uptake into body tissues of all the amino acids *except* tryptophan.

With the competition tied up, the tryptophan is free to attach itself to the carrier molecule and be transported to the brain, where it will then be converted into pain-relieving serotonin. *Easy plan:* Try a 10 percent protein, 10 percent fat, and 80 percent carbohydrate diet.

Where to Find Tryptophan

Your simplest method is to take *three* doses of 500 milligrams each, with your three daily meals. *Remember:* Your meals should be high-carb, low-fat, low-protein.

Food Sources: Included are milk, peanuts, eggs, and some meats. The last two items are high in cholesterol and fat, so you would have to restrict their intake.

It will be more effective if you take the supplements on a daily basis, reducing potency as the pain is reduced. If you anticipate a pain-causing stressful situation, be sure to take your tryptophan in advance to shield yourself against reactions.

HEALS STIFF NECK, ENDS NIGHTMARISH MIGRAINE HEADACHES,
CORRECTS BAD BACK WITH NUTRITIONAL THERAPY

JoAnne T. was a victim of excruciatingly tight stiff neck and frequent migraines that would last for days and nights. Her back was often hunched up, and she could never remember being able to walk or sit with a flexible spinal column. Nauseous and weak from medications, she was often bed-ridden until the attack was over.

Was this going to be her lifetime disability? She appealed for help from an osteopathic physician who diagnosed her condition as being tryptophan deficient to an alarming degree. He prescribed 1,500 milligrams per day, to be taken on a low-protein program. Within six days, her stiff neck was swanlike in flexibility, her headaches vanished, and she could move her shoulders with the agility of a dancer. What was erroneously said to be a "lifetime" affliction with pain was healed with nutritional therapy of tryptophan!

Suggestions, Hints, Programs

For quick-acting results, consider taking 500 milligrams of tryptophan on an empty stomach so it does not have to compete with other amino acids and can increase relaxing serotonin levels more rapidly. For some people, tryptophan taken at bedtime elevates serotonin enough to relax pains and increase ability to fall asleep all the more easily.

Avoid refined sugar in your diet. It influences brain serotonin levels by interfering with transfer of tryptophan into the brain.

You may take tryptophan with a fresh citrus fruit or juice which is a concentrated source of vitamin C. This nutrient works with tryptophan to block pain-causing impulses that threaten to hurt the neurons (brain cells). It is vitamin C that enables the tryptophan to cross the blood/brain barrier or impenetrable wall of tissues. Here, it blocks dopamine receptors or substances that are responsible for the pain.

In particular, vitamin C plus tryptophan have an affinity with the dopamine receptors, these two nutrients are able to help shield your brain (and body) from various types of pain.

Simple Nutritional Therapy Heals Pain
Swiftly

Just take a 500 milligram tablet of tryptophan with one glass of freshly prepared citrus juice. This is the powerful all-natural combination that will instantly send forth a supply of pain blockers and serotonin to heal the distress—and prevent it from happening again!

With the use of various nutritional therapies, you can look forward to living *without* your "incurable" pain. If need be, take two "nutrients" in the morning and see if you need to ask for medications the next day, or ever again!

SUMMARY

1. Medications with their temporary effects and extended side effects are not the only answer to correcting pain.
2. Phenylalanine is a nutritional amino acid that works as an all-natural pain killer.
3. Jim R. freed himself from years of headaches and stubborn pains with the use of a phenylalanine food supplement.
4. Magnesium is a soothing mineral that corrects the cause of muscular pain, unties knots, and eases the spasms in minutes.
5. Peggy MacD. kicked her "aspirin addiction" with the use of a Magnesium Tonic and freed herself of recurring pain within 1 hour.
6. Cool off your burning stress-caused pain with calcium.
7. Simple calcium snacks helped Benjamin X. to avoid pain attacks.
8. Tryptophan is a remarkable pain blocker that creates a protective barrier right in your brain cells to give you freedom from distress.
9. JoAnne T. overcame a lifetime threat of painful stiffness within six days with the use of tryptophan as nutritional therapy.

13

Sweeten Your Blood Sugar to Feel Youthful...in Minutes

Hypoglycemia, translated into lay terms, simply means low blood sugar. *Hypo* means low; *glycemia* means sugar. (Diabetes is the opposite: high blood sugar, or hyperglycemia.) Both conditions, while virtually opposite, are closely related. Both are caused by the body's inability to use sugar effectively.

Low Blood Sugar = Low Body and Mind Energy

In almost all persons who have low blood sugar, the most prominent symptom is fatigue of body and mind. You know you have this syndrome if you feel tired much of the time. That is, tired without obvious reason, tired when you awaken, often too tired to function effectively in household, occupational, or marital activities.

Warning Symptoms

These include emotional upset, irritability, difficulty in concentrating, muscle aches, weight gain, weak libido, recurring headaches, and, often, intolerance of even small amounts of alcohol.

Feel Depressed?

Mild to moderate depression is often traced to either a sudden drop in blood sugar or a seesaw "yank" that could give you feelings of elation one minute, then plunge you downward into the depths of the glooms the next. This disturbance of body chemistry known as hypoglycemia can sap away your vital energy even in the prime of life.

What Causes Hypoglycemia?

Hypoglycemia is a condition brought on by an insufficient amount of glucose (sugar) in the bloodstream. The villain here is sugar. It is like a firecracker. It agitates the brain chemistry. It incites the explosive behavior classified as hyperactive.

What happens is that the pancreas (a small gland lying behind the stomach) is overstimulated by sugar and secretes an overabundance of insulin, which reduces the sugar level in blood to a below-normal amount. Unless your blood has a proper level of sugar, your brain cannot function efficiently.

Constant overconsumption of sweets can undermine the biological mechanisms balancing blood sugar levels. This upset leads to erratic behavior, poor concentration, attention weakness, poor memory, and more physical signs such as a pale skin, premature aging, susceptibility to infections, and illness.

So-called Senility Could Be Hypoglycemia

The maintenance of a balanced blood sugar level is essential to achieving the best molecular environment for the mind. Hypoglycemia could bring on symptoms of so-called senility in which there are memory blanks, feelings of lethargy, staring off into space, inability to participate in ordinary conversations, feelings of confusion, and loss of identity. Many of these conditions have been sparked by the up-and-down "yo-yo" reaction of blood sugar. There could be feelings of exhilaration and energy that are soon changed to those of aging and disorientation. Your body is trying to signal the condition of hypoglycemia or low blood sugar.

Blood Sugar: Normal Versus Abnormal

Normally, the concentration of sugar or glucose in the blood is between 70 and 120 milligrams per 100 milliliters (mg/dl) before meals. Even with prolonged fasting, the blood glucose concentrations remains above 50 mg/dl. After meals, it may reach 140 for a short time, only to settle back down toward the premeal level. Hypoglycemia may be defined as a blood glucose concentration below 50 mg/dl, which may be considered "abnormal."

Your Body Must Have Sugar

You would not want to eliminate all forms of sugar from your diet. Neither could you, since it is found in almost everything you eat and drink. Your body uses glucose for a variety of biochemical functions. Your brain, for example, could not function for more than 3 minutes without glucose. You would age and wither away without sugar. Then where does the problem occur?

Sugar Metabolism at a Glance

To supply your needs, your liver manufactures glucose from ingested protein as the raw material for synthesis. When starches or dietary sugars are consumed, insulin is released from your pancreas in response to the rising blood sugar as the dietary carbohydrates are absorbed. Insulin restrains liver production of the sugar. The released insulin shuts down liver glucose output and a simultaneous tissue consumption of glucose.

These two actions control the rising blood glucose after meals and return it promptly to normal. Between meals, insulin secretion is reduced. This permits liver glucose production to resume so that even with protracted fasting, your blood glucose will not fall too low to provide brain function.

This finely tuned system provides your brain with sufficient glucose even between meals; there is regulation of your blood sugar content so that it does not drop too low (hypoglycemia or low blood sugar) or go too high (hyperglycemia or diabetes).

Why Sugar Metabolism Goes Wrong and How to Protect Yourself

To remain youthful in body and mind, sugar is needed for all muscle actions, especially for brain and nerve function. Stored glycogen is reconverted into a usable form, glucose, and transported by the blood to areas where it is needed.

Thus, when you eat sugar in the form of *natural* carbohydrates, your blood and tissues usually absorb only the amount of sugar needed for normal function.

Problem: When you eat food with *refined,* white, commercially produced sugar, the small molecule carbohydrates of these foods are absorbed quickly—sometimes almost instantaneously through the membranes of the mouth and stomach—causing a sudden flood of glucose into the bloodstream.

Such a flood of excess sugar into the bloodstream exerts a dangerous strain on the pancreas and liver, as well as the adrenals and other endocrine glands involved in regulating blood sugar levels. The firecracker explodes and hypoglycemia ignites the system.

So you can see that wholesome *natural* carbohydrates such as fresh fruits, vegetables, grains, and legumes can be metabolized to provide a steady supply of healthy sugar. But the *refined* carbohydrates such as white sugar, white flour, and processed and sugar-saturated packaged foods cause an overreactive pancreas that produces too much insulin. Blood sugar level drops abnormally low, depriving your brain and nervous system of much needed oxygen.

The sugar metabolism process goes haywire, and you suffer the penalty of unpleasant hypoglycemic symptoms.

Eating Sugar Is Like Throwing Fat on Fire

You would erroneously assume that to correct low blood sugar, just eat sugar! This is dangerous! Pouring in more sugar will only trigger your overresponsive pancreas to produce more insulin and worsen both the situation and the symptoms. The excess of refined sugars and carbohydrates will cause internal upheaval and explosive reactions just as throwing fat on a fire makes the fire worse. So it is with sugar as a remedy. The "cure" is worse than the disease!

"But I Don't Eat Sugar!"

Many a diagnosed functional hypoglycemia patient insists on never touching sugar so how can the condition develop? The answer is in "hidden" sugar. Nearly all soft drinks contain sugar. Many commonly used sauces, jellies, custards, canned fruits, or juices contain sugar. Virtually all canned, processed, frozen, or packaged foods contain some form of sugar additive. For example, all commercially sold bread contains sugar or syrup. *Read the label!*

Did you know that many frozen TV dinners whether meat, fish, dairy, fruit, or vegetable will also have sugar? These processed foods with so much concentrated sugar can easily overtax the pancreas and trigger its overreaction. So even if you never use the sugar bowl or shaker, but eat processed foods, you are also eating sugar! Therefore, to protect yourself against hypoglycemia, you would need to shun all forms of sugar, whether added by yourself or the cook or in processed foods.

Simple Corrective Program Shields You from Hypoglycemia

To guard against the risk of age-causing and allergy-inducing hypoglycemia, follow this simple five-step corrective and protective program:

1. *Avoid sugar.* A diet too high in refined starches and sugars will trigger hypoglycemia. Much of today's irrational and antisocial behavior can be traced to our denatured, chemicalized, sugar-laden diet. To eliminate these two health destroyers, use a rule of thumb to *avoid prepared* foods and drinks. Prepare your own from scratch. You will help stabilize your insulin production and guard against the tug of war threat of refined carbohydrates.

2. *Avoid caffeine.* Studies demonstrate that caffeine raises blood sugar level in diabetics, but drastically lowers it in hypoglycemics. This is not as contradictory as it may seem. Sugar does the same because of an overreacting pancreas. Caffeine has a stimulating effect on the adrenal glands, which prompt the liver to release more sugar into the bloodstream. Excessive caffeine produces such hypoglycemic symptoms as anxiety, light-headedness, heart palpitations, nervousness, agitation, irritability, trembling hands and muscle twitches, and sleep disorders. Caffeine is found in more products than just coffee (see chart 13-1). For most people, just 100 milligrams a day can trigger disorders. Just stop consuming caffeine-containing products, and the symptoms should vanish.

3. *Avoid alcohol.* Consider the condition of alcohol-induced hypoglycemia, for example, the "morning after" or the typical hang-over. These are little more than symptoms of hypoglycemia. Alcohol reduces the output of glucose by the liver, which then precipitates or exaggerates low blood sugar. Alcohol may well produce the same effect as sugar. To protect against this disorder, avoid alcohol just as you would avoid sugar.

4. *Avoid tobacco.* Some studies show that smoking will cause an abrupt rise in blood sugar and then a sudden drop when the cigarette or

Chart 13-1A: CAFFEINE CONTENT OF POPULAR BEVERAGES AND FOODS

Item	Milligrams of Caffeine
Coffee (5-ounce cup)	
Drip method	110–150
Percolated	64–124
Instant	40–103
Decaffeinated	2–5
Instant decaffeinated	2
Tea (loose or bags) (5-ounce cup)	
1 minute brew	9–33
3-minute brew	20–46
5-minute brew	20–50
Tea products	
Instant tea (5-ounce cup)	12–28
Iced tea (12-ounce can)	22–36
Cocoa	
Made from mix	6
Milk chocolate (1 ounce)	6
Baking chocolate (1 ounce)	35

Source: Data for caffeine content obtained from Consumers Union, Food and Drug Administration, National Coffee Association, and National Soft Drink Association.

13-1B: CAFFEINE CONTENT OF VARIOUS SOFT DRINKS

Soft Drinks with Caffeine	Milligrams of Caffeine (per 12 ounce serving)
Sugar-Free Mr. PIBB	58.8
Mountain Dew	54.0
Mello Yello	52.8
TAB	46.8
Coca-Cola	45.6
Diet Coke	45.6

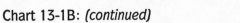

Chart 13-1B: *(continued)*

Soft Drinks with Caffeine	Milligrams of Caffeine (per 12 ounce serving)
Shasta Cola	44.4
Shasta Cherry Cola	44.4
Shasta Diet Cola	44.4
Shasta Diet Cherry Cola	44.4
Mr. PIBB	40.8
Dr. Pepper	39.6
Sugar-Free Dr. Pepper	39.6
Big Red	38.4
Sugar-Free Big Red	38.4
Pepsi-Cola	38.4
Aspen	36.0
Diet Pepsi	36.0
Pepsi Light	36.0
RC Cola	36.0
Diet Rite	36.0
Kick	31.2
Canada Dry Jamaica Cola	30.0
Canada Dry Diet Cola	1.2

*There are at least 68 flavors, variets, and types of soft drinks, manufactured by the 12 leading bottlers, that contain no caffeine.

Source: Data obtained from the National Soft Drink Association, Washington, D.C.

13-1C: CAFFEINE IN DRUG PREPARATIONS

Classification	Milligrams per tablet or capsule	Milligrams per day*
Over-the-counter		
Stimulants		
NoDoz tablets	100	200
Vivarin tablets	200	200
Pain relievers		
Anacin	32	64

Chart 13-1C: *(continued)*

Classification	Milligrams per tablet or capsule	Milligrams per day*
Excedrin	65	130
Midol	32	64
Plain aspirin, any brand	0	0
Vanquish	33	66
Diuretics		
Aqua-Ban	100	200
Cold remedies		
Coryban-D	30	30
Dristan	16.2	32.4
Triaminicin	30	30
Weight-control aids		
Dexatrim	200	200
Dietac	200	200
Prolamine	140	140
Prescription		
Cafergot	100	100
Darvon Compound	32.4	64.8
Fiorinol	40	40 or 80
Migrol	50	50

*Depending on the type of drug, a single dose is recommended nce a day or as often as once every four hours.

Source: Information on caffeine content and standard dosages obtained from the *Physicians' Desk Reference*, 1982, and *The Physicians' Desk reference for Nonprescription Drugs*, 1982.

cigar is put out. This rapid rise and fall of blood sugar levels also leads to the habit of chain smoking—the craving for another pick-me-up. This upset in the sugar control mechanism can cause emotional instability, apprehension, and insecurity along with typical physical disorders. Get rid of smoking, and you may well get rid of the risk of hypoglycemia.

5. *Avoid salt.* This additive causes a loss of blood potassium, which leads to a drop in blood sugar. You need potassium, a vital mineral,

to balance sugar metabolism. Yet excessive salt consumption disturbs this level, causing much potassium to be lost while sodium is retained in the system (known as edema or water retention). The connection between salt and hypertension, kidney malfunction, and cardiovascular disorders is well known. Kick the salt habit and you may kick the problem of erratic blood sugar.

Just build this five-step nutritional therapeutic program into your daily life-style and enjoy much more emotional and physical well-being.

RECOVERS FROM "OLD AGE" IN TWO DAYS ON EASY FIVE-STEP PROGRAM

George DeB. was losing his grip. Although only in his fifties, he walked with a stoop, looked with glazed eyes at once familiar family and friends, would be irritable for a few hours, then silently depressed for the next hours. He grew allergic to modest weather changes and exhibited faulty memory and slurred speech. Simple tasks were impossible. When he could not remember his address, concerned family worried he might be developing Alzheimer's disease or so-called senile old age.

Fortunately, an endocrinologist was consulted who diagnosed his condition as erratic blood sugar, responsible for his declining condition. George DeB. was put on the preceding five-step program. Nothing else! Within two days, he recovered so much, he was more alert mentally and physically than his grandson! He was cheerful, sharp in eyes and talk, resisted illnesses, had an alert mind, and was as cheerful as could be. The five-step program saved him from a "living death" of confinement in an institution with Alzheimer's disease!

How Simple Meal Spacing Gives You Superenergy and Vitality

Your goal is to normalize your metabolism. You can do this by following simple meal-spacing programs to give you day-long vitality of mind and body. Here are the easy-to-follow steps:

1. *Have a protein breakfast.* Start your day off with an energy bank in the form of protein. It is found in meats, fish, eggs, dairy products, beans, nuts, seeds, and whole grains. If you are watching your fat and/or cholesterol levels, just switch to egg whites or skim milk products. A good protein breakfast does not overload your blood with sugar but

sends glucose first to your liver, which doles out the sugar allowance as needed. This prevents overloading and subsequent bankruptcy of sugar in the bloodstream. *Caution:* The working person's typical breakfast of coffee and a sweet roll is definitely out! *Suggestion:* A fruit salad with a sprinkling of chopped nuts and seeds, some chunks of cheese, with a caffeine-free beverage is a good protein breakfast to give you day-long vigor.

2. *Take frequent meals.* If possible, have five or six meals instead of three traditional large ones. *Benefit:* By eating frequently, you consume less, and instead of having three wide upward and downward swings in blood sugar level, you have six or seven small ones. In time the level will tend to smooth out. A bonus is that small meals minimize conversion of food into fat and frequent meals control your appetite.

3. *Enjoy some fat.* Your nutritional therapy program calls for a small amount of dietary fat. It has satiety value that keeps away hunger pangs and also helps stoke the fires to burn body fat. Just 2 tablespoons of polyunsaturated vegetable oil daily on your salad or in cooking will help to balance your blood sugar, too.

4. *Surrender to the snack attack.* Your blood sugar is misbehaving and needs controls with the use of a good protein snack. Try a handful of sunflower seeds, a tablespoon of nutmeats, a half cup of salt-free, butter-free popcorn, a small portion of very lean meat, a fat-trimmed drumstick, a wedge of cheese with a slice of fruit. Just eat a *small* portion, perhaps a mouthful or two at the most. It will soon help your body utilize amino acids and carbohydrates and calm down your disruptive blood sugar.

5. *Never skip meals.* Skipping meals causes stored fat to pour into your bloodstream and poses a risk to your heart. Also, there is a confusion with carbohydrate metabolism that could trigger hypoglycemic symptoms. Once you plan your daily five- or six-meal schedule, stick to it. You will find yourself looking and feeling younger and healthier with a stabilized blood sugar level.

With this five-step program of meal spacing, you should quicky experience a return to normal blood sugar. You will feel it in the form of superenergy and vitality. And youthfulness, too!

FROM "WACKY" TO "WONDERFUL" IN FOUR DAYS

Her life was falling apart! Marion O'C. had worked for more than 15 years as a company supervisor with nary a personality problem, but now she was losing control. She snapped at coworkers. Columns of figures were confusing. Schedules were disrupted. She forgot to give messages to her superiors. Important papers were never prepared. Meetings were in disarray. Her antagonistic attitude dubbed her "wacky" by coworkers behind her back. What went wrong? Was she ready for discharge or, worse, confinement?

A sympathetic saleswoman recalled her sister having undergone a personality change to be diagnosed as hypoglycemic. When the family endocrinologist suggested regular spaced-out meals and avoidance of sugar, salt, and caffeine as part of a program of more natural foods, the symptoms vanished. She urged Marion O'C. to follow the same home treatment. Sneering, the emotionally unstable woman mumbled her doubts, yet she did follow the program. Within four days, she was cheerful again, mentally alert, and a superwhiz in efficiency. Her blood sugar had stabilized with the back-to-basics program, and she was now called "wonderful" by adoring coworkers.

Nutritional Therapies to Sweeten Your Blood Sugar

Your goal is to stabilize your blood sugar, or "sweeten" it. Obviously, without the use of inflammatory sugar. You can do it with a few nutrients that are known for correcting the functional imbalance and restore mental and physical equilibrium in a short time. In effect, these nutrients sweeten your blood sugar.

Chromium

A trace element needed for proper sugar metabolism. A deficiency can cause impairment of the sugar regulating machinery which is controlled by insulin. Chromium is needed to manufacture the glucose tolerance factor (GTF), whic regulates the blood sugar. *Food sources:* Included here are brewer's yeast, whole grains, wheat germ, and bran.

Zinc

Plentiful in a healthy pancreas where insulin is manufactured and is actually a constituent of that hormone. Those who are diagnosed as having hypoglycemia and/or diabetes are often found to be deficient in zinc. *Food sources:* Consider whole grains, seeds, and nuts.

Vitamins B-Complex

The entire B-complex family is helpful because they build your body's tolerance to sugars and carbohydrates and assist in promoting a more normal sugar metabolism. *Food sources:* Enjoy whole grains, brewer's yeast, green leafy vegetables, eggs, organ meats, nut butters, and brown rice.

Pantothenic Acid

A deficiency could cause blood sugar to drop so quickly, there could be a blackout or total collapse. This particular B-complex member is singled out because it is very intimately involved in the metabolism, synthesis, and breakdown of carbohydrates, fatty acids, sterols, and steroid hormones, all of which are involved in maintaining a balanced sugar level. *Food sources:* Try brewer's yeast, wheat germ, wheat bran, whole grain breads and cereals, beans, nuts, peas, liver, egg yolk, and green vegetables.

Magnesium

Magnesium is a nutritive substance that is required for blood sugar stabilization. It activates those enzyme systems that control fat and electrolyte metabolism. Low magnesium levels seem to be related to reactive hypoglycemia (a condition in which blood sugar drops precipitously following a meal rich in refined carbohydrates)—leaving the victim with symptoms of weakness, shakiness, dizziness, headache, irritability, and confusion, to name a few penalties. *Food sources:* Include in your diet whole grains, green leafy vegetables, beet greens, nuts, brown rice, and soybeans.

Quick Help for Boosting Blood Sugar

To give your blood sugar a "shot in the arm," you could try this easy to prepare Energy Shake because that is precisely what it does. It gives your sugar a lift and your body and mind an energy shake-up!

How to Prepare

Blenderize the following ingredients in an 8 or 10 ounce glass: 1 tablespoon brewer's yeast, 2 tablespoons wheat germ, 1 tablespoon sunflower seeds, 1 tablespoon nutmeats, 1 cup torn greens, 6 ounces skim milk. Whiz for just 2 or 3 minutes. Drink slowly.

Benefits: The chromium stimulates the manufacture of the GTF to balance your blood sugar. A flow of energy boosted by the zinc and B-complex vitamins along with the metabolic power of pantothenic and magnesium will send a supercharge of vitality throughout your endocrine system. Within 10 minutes, the Energy Shake corrects your glucose metabolic levels and you have swept away fog from your mind and knots from your muscles. You become revived, regenerated, refreshed—and rejuvenated!

Include These Foods on a Daily Basis

When planning your food program, be sure to include the foods already listed. They give you the valuable nutrients that are nonsystemic in that they zero in directly on those specific body and glandular areas needing their help.

BANISHES HEADACHES, IMPROVES MEMORY, BECOMES ENERGETIC IN JUST TWO DAYS

Edward L. had more than stubborn headaches and memory lapses. He felt his energy slipping through his fingers. He feared getting old before his time even though he was only in his early fifties. A diet specialist said he could have hypoglycemia. He recommended the easy-to-prepare Energy Shake. Edward L. had the shake in the morning; he also gave up all forms of refined sugars and starches as well as caffeine. Within two days, his headaches were gone, his memory was sharp, and he was a bundle of energy. His blood sugar had been stabilized, thanks to the program and the tasty and speedily effective beverage!

How a Glass of Milk Can Balance Your Sugar Levels

For many folks troubled with hypoglycemia, milk is a remarkably effective form of nutritional therapy. If you drink one glass of milk first thing in the morning and last thing at night, you could overcome your disorders. *Benefit:* Milk is rich in protein and also contains a small amounts of natural sugar (lactose), which very gently raises your blood sugar levels.

If you are calorie and fat cautious, drink low-fat or fat-free milk. You may very well eliminate the syndrome of low blood sugar with this simple nutritional therapy.

Are you a victim of hypoglycemia? Troubled with indecision, irritability, headaches, anxiety, digestive upsets? You may be a victim of hypoglycemia, an affliction called the "hidden disease" because its symptoms mimic other organic problems. With the use of nutritional therapy, you should put some sweetness into your body and mind and feel youthful, in minutes.

IN REVIEW

1. Check over the reasons why hypoglycemia happens and see if you fit into that diagnostic picture.
2. Note the differences between refined and natural sugars and carbohydrates and plan to avoid those foods that are processed.
3. Follow the five-step nutritional therapeutic program to shield yourself from the upset of low blood sugar.
4. George DeB. went from "old age" to youth in two days with the easy five-step program.
5. Simple meal spacing helps to improve your natural energy reserves.
6. Using the improved meal plan program, Marion O'C. went from hypoglycemic "wacky" to healthy "wonderful" in four days.
7. Include the nutrient-rich foods in your meal planning, as listed, to improve sugar metabolism.
8. Easy to prepare, an Energy Shake works in minutes like a "shot in the arm" to give you a mind-body boost.
9. Edward L. was "restored to life" with the basic dietary improvements and the Energy Shake that worked instantly.
10. For many cases of sugar imbalance, a glass of milk twice daily may well be the most potent (and easiest) nutritional therapy you need to put you in the pink and correct your low blood sugar.

14

For Men Only: Solve Prostate Problems with Nutritional Therapy

If you are a male over age 50, has this ever happened to you? After driving for miles and miles, the need to go to a rest stop keeps building until the pressure seems uncontrollable. Relief is in sight when you approach a gas station. You know where your bladder is located. It is at that point in the lower abdominal cavity where you felt all that unbearable pressure.

The problem is not necessarily with your bladder, partially responsible for your having to make increasing bathroom trips, especially during the night. Instead, there could be a disorder with your prostate gland.

Location, Function of Prostate

This walnut-sized organ is located next to the bladder (where urine is stored) and surrounds the urethra (canal through which urine passes out of the body). The prostate manufactures the liquid that acts as a vehicle for the sperm cells. During sexual activity, it secretes fluid to transport sperm into the vagina for the purpose of fertilizing the female's egg and fulfill the normal process of reproduction. Without the prostate gland to manufacture this essential fluid, the male becomes sterile.

Normal Versus Abnormal Prostate Gland

A normal walnut-sized prostate can be pictured as a bunch of tiny grapelike bulbs, fitting snuggly around the urethra so it can empty prostatic fluid into that tube at the moment of orgasm. The abnormal enlarged prostate puts restricting pressure on the urethra, increasing the time it takes to empty the bladder. The more the prostate enlarges, the greater is the pressure and the more difficult it becomes to get the bladder completely empty.

Is Your Prostate Giving You a Hard Time?

Be alert to these early warning signals of an enlarged or inflamed prostate (prostatitis)—a feeling of congestion and discomfort in the pubic area. You have a constant feeling of fullness of the bladder, with frequent, desperate trips to the bathroom. Often, there is difficulty in being able to void; sometimes there is no passage at all.

The recurring need to void during the night is distressingly common. It disturbs your sleep. Eventually, waste residue collects in the bladder, and some release is possible. The difficulty can be serious if the urethra is so blocked that little can be discharged from the bladder. The risk of uremic poisoning arises when your bladder is overloaded with fluid. With the normal avenue of release through the urethra blocked off, waste floods back into the kidneys, presenting a serious danger of poison to your system.

Be Alert to Seven Warning Symptoms

Prostate difficulties should not be taken lightly or ignored in the hope that they will just go away. There is the constant danger that the ailing prostate will enlarge and constrict the urethra and impede or completely block the passage of urine. Such a condition can be extremely painful and even fatal if not treated. Here is a checklist of warning signals that indicate you need to visit your health practitioner for a prostate examination:

1. Low back pain.
2. Blood in the urine or in the seminal fluid.
3. An increase in sexual excitability or frequent erections that come without any special stimulation.
4. Pain during the ejaculation of the seminal fluid.
5. Impotence or premature ejaculation.
6. A chronic sense of fullness in the bowel and difficulty in passage of waste.
7. Any loss in control over urination, such as difficulty in starting or stopping the stream or inability to slow the stream.

Even if you feel confident there is nothing wrong with your prostate, you should have an accurate medical diagnosis of any difficulty. You could be saving your prostate gland from disease or removal!

Common Prostate Problems

Acute prostatitis is a bacterial infection that can occur in men at any age. Symptoms include fever, chills, and painful or difficult urination; also pain in the lower back and between the legs.

Chronic prostatitis is a recurring infection. Symptoms are similar to those of acute prostatitis but usually milder. If no disease-causing infectious bacteria are found, massaging of the prostate helps to release blocked-up fluids.

Benign prostatic hypertrophy (BPH) is an enlargement of the prostate. It is caused by small noncancerous tumors that grow inside the prostate. They are believed to be related to hormone changes with aging. The enlarged prostate may eventually obstruct the urethra and cause difficulty in urinating, along with urges during the night.

Prostate cancer, occurring mainly in men over age 60, is third in the number of new cancer cases in men each year (76,000) and third in deaths (25,000). A regular rectal exam, especially for men over 40, helps to detect prostate cancer, and the five-year relative survival rate is 75 percent, if found early and treated promptly. In the early stages of prostate cancer, the disease stays localized (in the prostate) and does not endanger life. But without treatment, the cancer can spread to other tissues and eventually cause fatality. Prostate cancer usually progresses very slowly. When symptoms do appear, they are usually similar to those caused by BPH.

A urologist (a specialist in disorders of the urinary system) is often recommended as a qualified doctor to diagnose and treat the prostate.

Protecting Yourself

The best protection against prostate problems is to have regular medical checkups that include a thorough and careful prostate exam. See your health practitioner promptly if unusual symptoms occur, such as a frequent urge to void or difficulty in passing wastes. Waiting until severe symptoms appear may result in serious and sometimes life-threatening complications.

How Zinc Is Able to Keep Your Prostate
in Its Prime

To prolong and extend the health of your prostate, zinc is a major form of nutritional therapy. The prostate accumulates high levels of zinc, more than any other organ of the body. It has also been noted that when there is benign hypertrophy of the prostate, there is a deficiency of zinc. In conditions of chronic prostatitis, which has not only enlargement but infection, the zinc concentration is lowest of all. This mineral is also involved in proper sperm function, sexual health, and several basic reproductive hormone systems.

The importance of zinc to the prostate is reflected in the fact that this gland contains a concentration of this mineral some 10 times greater than most other organs of the body. Zinc has a unique influence on the swimming ability of sperm, which must be strong enough to reach a woman's fallopian tubes and penetrate the egg for fertilization to take place.

An adequate amount of serum (blood) zinc levels is believed able to protect against disorders of the prostate and also correct such problems in a short time. Many laboratory investigations have shown that zinc is able to protect the prostate against deterioration.

Food Sources of Prostate-Nourishing Zinc

These include brewer's yeast, nuts, eggs, rice bran, onions, chicken, beans, peas, lentils, wheat germ, wheat bran, beef liver, and gelatin. Some of these sources (eggs, chicken, beef liver) may be too high in fat and cholesterol so you would want to opt for the other foods. Zinc supplements are available at health stores and pharmacies; a general rule of thumb is to take 35 milligrams per day as a means of building resistance to disorders and easing symptoms. Your health practitioner can give you specific guidelines for your needs.

SHRINKS ENLARGED PROSTATE WITH NUTRITIONAL THERAPY

His urologist confirmed that Nicholas L. was facing enlargement of the prostate gland. Urinary difficulties compounded with pain spasms had alerted him to this disorder. Fortunately, he appeared for help in the early stages of benign prostatic hypertrophy (BPH) so he was able to avoid surgery with its attendant risks. His treatment consisted of boosting blood levels of zinc. He was told to increase intake of whole grains and legumes (see preceding food source list) and also to take 35 milligrams of zinc as a supplement each day. Within 16 days, his prostate gland started to shrink. He no longer had to get up repeatedly throughout the night. His voiding was with no discomfort. At the end of 30 days, his urologist informed him that the simple, but effective, nutritional therapy of zinc had given him a normal-sized prostate again, along with a feeling of youth!

How Zinc Helps to Zap Prostate Infections

Zinc zeroes in to act as a catalyst (helper) in many biological reactions to nourish and rejuvenate your prostate gland. Zinc gathers a number of nutrients, especially amino acids, and uses them to knit and repair the delicate tissues and tubules of your prostate to keep it in youthful function. Zinc plays a vital role in carbohydrate metabolism so that sources of energy are built into your prostate to keep it alive, healthy, and young. Zinc helps to detoxify bacterial infections and knock out the virus invaders that could lead to infections of this male gland. So to keep your prostate in working condition at any age: think zinc!

Zinc Drink for Prostate Power

You can easily prepare a power-packed Zinc Drink that will strengthen the infection-fighting resources of your prostate to keep it in a healthy state of life:

Combine 1 glass of skim milk, 2 tablespoons wheat germ, 1 tablespoon wheat bran, ½ cup cooked cowpeas (blackeye), and blenderize for just three minutes or until foamy. Sip slowly.

Benefits: The high potency of zinc will combine with the calcium and amino acids to join with the essential fatty acids to go directly to your prostate. In a matter of moments, this powerhouse of nutritional therapy will regenerate and "cleanse" your prostate and give it a new lease on life. Plan to have this easily prepared Zinc Drink at least once a day, and watch your body respond with prostate power in no time at all!

ZINC DRINKS WASHES AWAY PROSTATE PAIN IN THREE DAYS

When Daniel McK. was told by his urologist that he was showing symptoms of prostate enlargement, a reason for his pain when he had to make repeated trips to the bathroom, he asked about nutritional helps to nip the problem in the bud. Because his tests showed a simultaneous deficiency in zinc, his doctor recommended boosting intake of this mineral. He included the zinc-containing foods and also had one or two Zinc Drinks every day. Results? Almost overnight, with raised zinc levels, the pain and annoying frequent urination began to go away. Within two days, the pain was gone; his voiding was almost normal. The third day he felt "as good as new" and no longer complained of painful discomfort and frightening excessive urination. Zinc had washed away his prostate pain and restored fitness to his male gland—and entire body, too!

The "Magic" of Pumpkin Seeds for Prostate Fitness

You have probably enjoyed snacking on pumpkin seeds in the past. Chock full of vitamins and minerals, they are known for being a concentrated source of vegetable protein. But they also offer a "magic" source of *essential fatty acids,* which are gobbled up by your prostate gland as the very source of its life.

EFAs, as they are known, are important for helping to preserve the health, the virility, and the potency of your prostate. These nutrients, highly concentrated in pumpkin seeds, work with zinc to keep your delicate tubules, cells, and tissues in smooth working order. They enter right into the prostatic fluid to determine vigor and strength and overall fitness. Essential fatty acids include linoleic acid, linolenic acid, and arachidonic acid. These same EFAs are needed to carry vitamins A, D, E, and K to the prostate for overall nourishment.

Chew Pumpkin Seeds for Prostate Rejuvenation

Just a handful of pumpkin or sunflower seeds will give you a powerhouse of these prostate-rejuvenating essential fatty acids. You may also want to include safflower oil, corn oil, sunflower seed oil, wheat germ oil, soybean oil, and sesame seed oil. To nourish your prostate further with EFAs, try walnut meats, Brazil nuts, pine nuts, peanuts, pecans, and almonds. A rich concentrated source is wheat germ!

With these tasty forms of nutritional therapy, you should be able to give your prostate the rejuvenated power it needs to maintain overall youthfulness.

Vegetables Help to Rebuild Your Prostate

In a long-term study of 120,000 men, epidemiologists searched for some pattern in the dietary habits of those who had a significantly lower rate of prostate cancer. They found it!

The figures, they reported, "revealed a significantly lower age-standardized death rate for prostate cancer in men who daily ate *green and yellow vegetables*. This association is consistently observed in each age group, in each socioeconomic class, and in each prefecture or geographic area." The same scientists pointed out that other evidence supported this finding. Vegetarians living in the United States, such as Seventh-Day Adventists, have also been shown to have a lower risk of prostate cancer than the general population.

What, precisely, was the key prostate-saving element? Perhaps vitamin A, they suggested. But vegetables are also high in fiber (to speed up passage of wastes through the organ and reduce the amount of time carcinogens are in contact with cellular walls) as well as many vitamins and minerals. Vegetables are also low in fat. It is this combination of nutritional factors that would make green and yellow vegetables a powerful means of building and rebuilding prostate health.[1]

How Garlic Keeps Your Prostate Free of Infection

Volatile garlic is a powerhouse of *natural antibiotics* that help to insulate your prostate against the risk of infectious bacteria. A European electrobiologist, Professor Gurwitch, discovered that garlic releases a form of ultraviolet radiation called mitogenetic radiations. These emissions, now referred to as Gurwitch rays in the scientific world, have the ability of stimulating cell growth and activity of your prostate gland. Garlic would then appear to have this natural antibiotic property that would (1) shield your prostate against parasitic infections and (2) repair and reconstruct weakened glandular tissues so they give you a healthy organ.

Garlic is a prime source of allicin, a substance to help cleanse away decomposed bacteria that might otherwise cause prostatic infection.

[1]National Cancer Institute Monographs, No. 53, 1979.

Garlic possesses a powerful penetrative force. Within moments after being digested, the Gurwitch rays are able to uproot and discharge infectious bacteria and promote healing and regeneration of this vital male gland.

Had Your Garlic Today? Only your prostate will know! Just one or two cloves thoroughly chewed and swallowed with a vegetable juice will give you the inner protection against prostatic disorder. Or else dice several cloves in a green and yellow vegetable salad and add some pumpkin seeds along with just 1 tablespoon of a sesame seed oil for dressing.

This will give you a chewy good and tasty powerhouse of nutrients, bolstered with garlic, to strengthen your prostate and give you a "forever young" feeling.

Seven-Step Program for Prostate Health

This program will help to prevent prostate disorders and also improve the general health of this valuable male gland:

1. Practice moderation in marital relation. Do not go to any extremes. Enjoy your status as part of your picture of health.

2. Sexual excitation should have an ejaculation. Prolonged engorgement (blood accumulation) and suppressed or incomplete discharge may lead to functional and structure damage to your prostate gland.

3. Avoid smoking and drinking. Both can lead to the predisposition of prostate disorders.

4. Keep your general health status on a high level.

5. Keep yourself fit. Exercise daily. Walking is an excellent way to keep your prostate in good shape. Plan to devote 60 minutes per day to some beneficial exercise.

6. Make the most of nutritional therapies with the use of the nutrients described in this chapter.

7. Foods that promote a healthy prostate include raw pumpkin or sunflower seeds, cold-pressed vegetable oils, garlic, and essential fatty acids.
Regardless of your age, the earlier you take care of your prostate with nutritional therapy, the healthier it will be in years to come.

SUMMARY

1. Review the seven warning symptoms that reveal possible disorder of the prostate.

2. Zinc is a powerful mineral that keeps your prostate in its prime. Include food sources of this important mineral in your eating program throughout the week.

3. Nicholas L. helped to shrink his enlarged prostate with the use of his urologist-recommended zinc-boosting program.

4. For quick prostate protection, enjoy the power-packed Zinc Drink daily.

5. Daniel McK. was able to wash away prostate pain in three days with the tasty and effective Zinc Drink.

6. Pumpkin seeds have a "magic" prostate healer in the form of essential fatty acids.

7. Vegetables may be a key to prostate health and prevention of cancer.

8. Garlic is a natural antibiotic that builds prostate resistance to infection.

9. Follow the seven-step program for prostate health.

15

For Women Only: Foods to Soothe Monthly Tension and Ease the Change

A nutritional approach is able to help women cope with the difficulties encountered with the twin problems of, first, premenstrual syndrome or PMS and, second, the change of life or menopause. With the use of better nutrition and an adjustment in life-style, the glands become stabilized, and symptoms are eased, often eliminated. To understand how to use nutrition, let us take each of these difficulties on an individual basis.

Premenstrual Syndrome: Hormonal Roller Coaster

One major difference between a man's and a woman's body is that a woman's hormones are in a constant state of flux, while a man's sex hormones remain rather stable until called upon to function. When a woman of reproductive age feels that "mood indigo," she knows she is about to have her menstrual period. She is not alone!

The PMS Picture

Over 90 percent of women are said to admit having some form or degree of PMS. Estimates vary widely on how many women suffer significant emotional and physical symptoms. Some researchers claim 58 percent, while others report figures as low as 3 to 15 percent. About 10 percent require or seek treatment for their symptoms. It is generally believed that over 25 million women endure severe hormonal imbalance affecting them 10 days out of every month. Some become frightened by shocking fluctuations in mood, depression, and weight gain. These hormonal body changes are often misunderstood and this only adds to the distress. A smaller number of women report anger, nervousness, and food cravings. Common physical complaints are headache, bloating, fatigue, and insomnia.

What Causes PMS?

The precise causes are believed to be related to the hormonal cycle because symptoms and findings recur with such regularity. During the early part of each cycle, ovaries produce the female hormone called estrogen. After ovulation, a second hormone, progesterone is produced. This is essential for the health of any early pregnancy. It makes the lining of the uterus (endometrium) thicker, storing food and swelling the uterus. Also it causes general body tissues to retain more sodium from salt which draws more water and fluid into body tissue spaces causing swelling. Some PMS symptoms may be caused by this swelling in the uterus, pelvis, abdomen, legs, liver, or brain.

While some women can cope with mild forms of PMS, for others, the physical and emotional stress can be overwhelming. These women become frightened by violent fluctuations in mood, depression, and weight gain. They react with physical and emotional disorders. PMS can be upsetting to the women—and all those who are in her midst!

The Reason Why PMS Brings On Pain

Medical research has confirmed that menstrual cramps are caused by a body chemical called *prostaglandin*. This substance is always present in the lining of the uterus, but it is kept in check by the female hormone *progesterone*. This hormone is at a high level two weeks before your period because its duty is to help a nutrient-carrying blood supply reach your uterus each month. This uterine wall blood buildup is your body's way of preparing for pregnancy. As soon as your brain receives a signal, however, that the egg (ovum) which has dropped into the uterus lining during your ovulation cycle will not be fertilized, the progesterone level drops. This enables the prostaglandin to be released, so it can prompt the smooth muscles in the uterus to contract and push the blood lining out.

If your body has a high level of prostaglandin, your uterus will overcontract, bringing on pain, cramps, and bloated swelling. *Problem:* Some prostaglandin spills into the bloodstream to affect your involuntary smooth muscles (those over which you have no conscious control). These include muscles in your heart, blood vessels, intestines, and uterus. That is why you may experience headaches, backaches, nausea, diarrhea, dizziness, hot and cold flashes, and fever, along with the painful cramping.

Blame It on Your Prostaglandins

When these substances start to act up, they put you on a roller coaster of disorders that may be mild at one time of the day only to become more disruptive and upsetting at another time of the day. Small wonder that women feel such frustration and despair when the prostaglandins cause these biological changes for most of the 10 days each month.

How Nutrition Pampers Prostaglandins and Eases PMS Pain

A change in diet with improved nutritional therapy can soothe the raging prostaglandins and help chase PMS blues. To help you tame discomfort, the following home programs are of welcome relief.

Vitamin B₆ or Pyridoxine

This nutrient influences the release of your brain's neurotransmitters (dopamine and serotonin) to help stabilize your moods. Vitamin B₆ helps to ease the throbbing of the pain-causing prostaglandins, helping you ease your way through the monthly period. With this nutrient, there is a balancing release of the soothing neurotransmitters and the pain is either eased or just erased. *Potency:* Prior to your period, taking 5 to 10 milligrams of vitamin B₆ daily will help to reduce pain and also edema and act as a natural diuretic. The pyridoxine also helps to relieve depression caused by high estrogen levels. This vitamin acts as a natural antispasmodic. *Food sources:* Enjoy brewer's yeast, potatoes, salmon, vegetables, and unmilled whole grains such as breads and cereals. *Suggestion:* Because the B-complex vitamins act together in harmony, it would be helpful to take a multivitamin-mineral tablet with adequate pyridoxine. Include the foods in your daily plan for more nutritional therapy.

Calcium

Ten days prior to the period, calcium levels in your blood drop radically. This deficiency triggers depression, nervousness, severe muscle cramps, edema, and headaches. With calcium, the heart beats normally, and there is better nerve conduction, muscle contraction, hormone secretions. Calcium may well be a woman's "monthly friend" to help her breeze through PMS. *Potency:* From 1,000 to 1,500 milligrams daily will help to maintain a smoother muscular network. Because calcium works best when taken with magnesium, your plan should be to take both of these minerals together. To maintain a balance, the magnesium is taken at half the calcium intake. If you take 1,000 milligrams of calcium, then take 500 milligrams of magnesium at the same time. This is the effective ratio. *Food sources:* Calcium is found in milk, sardines, Gruyère cheese, cheddar cheese, and salmon. Magnesium is found in nuts, soybean seeds, whole grains, and green leafy vegetables such as chard, kale, and beet tops.

Zinc

During PMS, a zinc deficiency may lower your body's resistance to infection and impede your healing process. It may also lead to irritability, depression, and other symptoms such as headaches and nervousness. *Potency:* Your body will be soothed with 30 milligrams of zinc per day; it is best to take it along with calcium and magnesium but *not* with iron. When zinc and iron are combined, both minerals prevent each other's absorption into the bloodstream. *Food sources:* In varying amounts, it is found in meat, poultry, eggs, milk, and especially whole grains.

Potassium

This valuable mineral helps to regulate fluid retention. If you feel bloated, it could be traced to a potassium deficiency, which is to blame for retention of sodium and fluid in your cells. Potassium acts as an *electrolyte,* or spark plug, that helps to cast out sodium weight from your cells and control bloatedness. *Potency:* your daily requirement ranges from 1,875 to 5,625 milligrams. But since it is easily available in such a wide variety of foods, a supplement may not be required, except as prescribed by your health practitioner. *Food sources:* Consider bananas, oranges or orange juice, sun-dried fruits, and untoasted and unsalted nutmeats.

Vitamin E

This nutrient prevents oxidation of fatty substances such as vitamin E, essential fatty acids, and the adrenal, pituitary, and sex hormones. It is believed that vitamin E also guards against fibrocystic breast conditions and even promotes healing of this syndrome. To help establish hormonal balance, vitamin E would seem therapeutic. *Potency:* From 500 to 800 units daily. *Food sources:* Consider wheat germ, vegetable oils, nuts, whole grain breads, and cereals.

Tryptophan

As explained in Chapter 12, the amino acid tryptophan is needed to manufacture serotonin, one of the brain's mood regulators. It seems reasonable that if tryptophan is needed to create serotonin, and a serotonin deficiency brings on depression, then a woman should take tryptophan. This would change the "blue" mood that may be part of the syndrome. It is a personal reaction, and you can find out if it helps you only if you try it. *Potency:* If symptoms of PMS-induced depression are severe, you could begin with 500 milligrams of tryptophan a day and increase to 1,000 and then 1,500 until you feel relief. Each woman knows her disposition and senses her well-being. You can judge better than anyone else what amount of tryptophan seems to improve your condition. *Food sources:* Enjoy wheat bran, wheat germ, cooked soy beans, raw mushrooms.

Essential Fatty Acids

The newer scientific knowledge of nutrition and PMS points to EFAs as being most essential to maintain biological balance. PMS is believed to be triggered by a deficiency of these essential fatty acids, especially linoleic and linolenic acids. There are blocking factors that interfere with the absorption, uptake, and utilization of essential fatty acids. There is more glandular upheaval because the prostaglandins are upset without enough essential fatty acids. *Potency:* Approximately 5 to 6 grams daily are all you need—the amount found in just two teaspoons of any of these food sources available in everyday items. *Food sources:* Include safflower, sunflower, corn, wheat germ, soybean, and sesame seed oil. You may also obtain these EFAs in walnuts, Brazil nuts, pine nuts, peanuts, pecans, and hulled sunflower seeds.

Simple Tips to Ease PMS Distress

Nutritional therapy is the foundation for hormonal stabilization. Other methods of relief are:

1. *Avoid salt.* You need to prevent fluid retention by avoiding salt whether in foods or from the shaker. You will help to protect against weight gain and bloating.

2. *Avoid sugar.* Insulin overshoot as overproduction of insulin in response to a sugar load can give you a PMS "hang-over." A concentrated sugar dose is especially dangerous because it pulls the trigger that causes eruption of endocrine responses known as PMS. A particularly sensitive time is during the last half of the menstrual cycle. There are two changes: an imbalance of the brain's hormones and neurotransmitters and an imbalance in the female hormones (estrogen and progesterone), and this could cause a sugar craving. *Problem:* Cells bind insulin and create a high sugar level to create a blood sugar upheaval. The hormones are now "crazed" by the sugar reaction and symptoms set in. *Nutritional therapy:* Avoid refined sugar in any form for easing of PMS distress.

3. *Avoid caffeine.* It overstimulates the brain and affects the central nervous system, activity of the heart and circulatory system, affecting coordination and respiration. By changing a woman's metabolic rate, caffeine also creates an internal situation in which insulin increases, blood sugar drops, and a hypoglycemiclike attack occurs. Just avoid caffeine in coffee, tea, cola, and chocolate products. Many over-the-counter and prescribed medications also contain caffeine. Read labels. Discuss a caffeine-free product with your health practitioner.

Plan Ahead for Symptom-Free PMS

Remember that PMS begins as progesterone levels drop, about 10 days before the period. The drop should be gradual. But if you are under stress or are enduring severe emotional problems, you may have a rapid drop of the hormone and a more pronounced shock through your body and mind.

Plan ahead. At least 10 days before the approach of your next period include the nutritional therapeutic programs outlined to build resistance and health to meet the challenges ahead. Life-style and dietary measures are most effective in controlling what could be a menstrual monster!

Warmth and Exercise Offer
Natural Relief

Try to ease discomfort with these natural programs:

Warmth

Apply heat to a painful area. Place a heating pad or hot water bottle under your back or on your abdomen will help to relax your uterus and ease cramps and spasms.

Comfort-pose Exercise

Do this regularly. It helps to shrink fatty tissue, thereby lessening menstrual flow and lowering prostaglandin levels. Try this comfort pose: lie on your back. Slowly bring your knees up to your chest. Then clasp your knees with your hands and pull them toward your armpits. While in this position, move your feet in a circular motion. Within moments, you should feel the spasms yielding to an overall feeling of total body comfort. Just 10 minutes each morning (or evening) will help to ease cramps or pain.

NUTRITION RESCUES WOMAN FROM PMS ROLLER COASTER

Carol DiG. was a "witch" to live with. Family, friends, and coworkers (she was a programmer for a leading computer firm) tried to keep out of her way as soon as she entered her period. She was irritable, would yell for no reason, snap at long-time friends and family, and was a persistent complainer. At times, she would burst out into tears, for no apparent reason. She was alienating her family and others in her circle.

An insurance company endocrinologist came to the rescue. Identifying her disorder as PMS, she was told to take the various nutrients from foods or prescribed supplements. Carol DiG. also changed her eating plan to avoid salt, sugar, and caffeine in any form. Within a few days, her self-control had returned. Her smiling disposition returned. She breezed through the period with nary a symptom. Thanks to nutritional therapy, she put her body (and mind) back on the track and got right off the roller coaster that was turning her into a "witch."

Quick Helps to Relieve Symptoms

A natural analgesic (pain reliever) is possible with the use of quickly prepared health tonics. They work swiftly in helping to block the antagonistic action of pain-causing prostaglandins and help to establish hormonal tranquility.

Muscle Relaxant Tonic

In a blender, combine 1 banana, 6 ounces of skim milk, 1 tablespoon wheat germ, 1 teaspoon nutmeats, and 1 teaspoon brewer's yeast. Blenderize for 3 to 4 minutes or until thoroughly liquefied. Drink slowly. *Benefit:* The rich concentration of potassium, calcium and magnesium work with vitamins B_6 and E to help ease contractions that are responsible for muscular pains during the monthly cycle. Just one glass of the Muscle Relaxant Tonic will help you cope with PMS for several days.

Mood Improvement Mix

Blenderize 2 teaspoons brewer's yeast, 6 ounces of orange juice, 1 tablespoon wheat germ, 1 tablespoon vegetable oil, and 1 teaspoon nutmeats. When thoroughly liquefied, drink before breakfast. *Benefit:* To help control the neurotransmitters that release mood-soothing hormones, the vitamin B_6 with the potassium and magnesium work to help your brain cope with the monthly cycle to give you an elevated mood of cheerfulness. *Tip:* Drink early in the morning on an empty stomach so nutrients can work swiftly and without interference from other foods to help give you mental stability.

Midday Pickup

Combine 3 ounces of skim milk, 3 ounces of orange juice, 1 teaspoon brewer's yeast, 1 teaspoon wheat germ, 1 tablespoon vegetable oil, and several sun-dried fruits in a blender. Liquefy for just 3 to 4 minutes. Drink in midday or during your "coffee break" as a healthful substitute or even as a lunch-in-a-glass. *Benefit:* The rich concentration of calcium, vitamin B_6, potassium, as well as vitamin E and the spectrum of the B-complex family helps you snap back to alertness in midday, when you have duties and obligations to perform.

Suggestion: Prepare a thermos of either of these natural analgesic beverages. Take along with you if you have to be on the road or at work or out of the house. When you need a pain reliever or just want to feel better try this beverage. You will find yourself feeling better and happier in minutes.

SAY "GOODBYE" TO PMS WITH NATURAL PAIN RELIEVERS

Viola J. was tied up in painful knots when in the midst of her monthly cycle. She could feel agonizing spasms shooting through her midsection in the middle of the day when she had so many tasks to perform. Hot flushes and nervousness worsened the condition. Viola J. had taken patent remedies, but because they had caffeine and irritating chemicals, they left her more shaken than before.

A nutrition-minded gynecologist suggested she reach for any of the preceding all-natural pain relievers at the slightest spasm or threat of one. Viola J. prepared the beverages. She discovered that one glass of either beverage every day protected her against pain. She could actually "sail through" the monthly cycle without any distress signals. She boasted about saying "goodbye" to her formerly ache-filled syndrome because of the use of nutritional therapy in the beverages.

PMS is a biological fact of life. But you do *not* have to accept the suffering of premenstrual syndrome. You can use nutritional therapy to meet the challenges of the pain cycle and save your body and sanity, if not your life!

Menopause—It's Time for a Change

Menopause or "change of life" is the time in a woman's life when menstruation stops and the body no longer produces the monthly ovum or egg from which a baby could be formed. It usually occurs at about age 50, although it may occur as early as 45 or as late as 55 and in some cases even earlier or later. Approximately 1.5 million women will undergo menopause in an average year. Every woman who lives beyond middle age eventually experiences it.

Starting as early as when a woman is in her late twenties, the ovaries begin a gradual decline. They become less sensitive to gonadotropins—pituitary gland hormones from the brain. Consequently, the occasions when ovulation (egg production) fails become more frequent. Likewise, production of estrogens, the female hormones, by the ovaries gradually lessens.

The Glandular Involvement

Most women notice no change until age 40 or more. Thereafter, the pituitary gland tries to correct the decline in estrogens by secreting more gonadotropins, particularly the follicle-stimulating hormone (FSH). The extra FSH usually shortens the first half of the menstrual cycle by speeding development of the ova (egg). Thus, the first premenopausal sign most women observe is a shortening of the menstrual cycle.

When a woman enters the menopause or climacteric, generally in her mid- to late-forties, anovulatory cycles become common. That is, the ovaries produce no ovarian progesterone (a female hormone) to counter the estrogen-induced thickening of the uterine lining (endometrium). When estrogen falls at the end of that cycle, unusually heavy bleeding may follow. The ovaries are literally running out of egg-producing follicles. Menstrual cycles become irregular.

Eventually, the ovaries no longer respond at all. They produce no ova, no estrogen, no progesterone. The endometrium no longer builds up and sheds in a cyclical period. Menopause has occurred.

Symptoms That Trouble the Change of Life

With the change can come upsetting disorders that may make the woman wonder which is the lesser of two evils: PMS or the change? Both are facts of life. But they are not inevitable. With nutritional therapy to be described shortly, they can be troubles that are easily resolved. Common and uncommon symptoms include the following:

Hot flushes or "hot flashes" are due to the opening of small blood vessels in the skin which produce sensations of extreme heat with reddening, "flushing" of the body, sometimes followed by drenching sweats. There is a disorder of the brain's temperature control center. They may last just a few seconds or up to half an hour or longer. Hot flushes can occur several times during the day or night or once a week or less.

Depression wavers with transient states of emotional upheaval. Irritability, emotional lability (frequent, rapid mood swings), and periods of depression are most likely when estrogen drops very suddenly as happens during menopause. (Lack of sleep caused by hot flashes can exacerbate emotional stress.)

Thinning of the linings of vagina and urinary tract are noted five or more years after menopause. In nearly all women over 60, lack of estrogen hampers the restoration of tissues lining these areas. They become fragile, lose tone, and are easily torn or infected. Vaginitis (vaginal inflammation, itching, and discharge) is fairly common.

Osteoporosis or the loss of bone calcium results in bone thinning. They body skeleton becomes so brittle and fragile that bones can break spontaneously during bending, lifting, or even walking. The marrow cavities enlarge. Falls frequently result in breaks. Bones of the wrist, hip, and spine are most susceptible. Bones can erode at up to 3 percent a year in the first three years after menopause. Then the rate slows. Women with severe osteoporosis lose up to 30 percent of their bone mass by age 70. Noticeable loss of height or development of a "dowager's hump" occur only when osteoporosis is severe.

You can prepare for a healthy menopause. If you are now in the midst of the "change," you can use simple home programs to help you avoid or minimize the symptoms listed.

How to Cool Off Hot Flashes

A hot flash is due to vasomotor instability, which is a rapid change in the diameter of the blood vessels. Just be calm. The heat will be over in less than 2 minutes. It will run its course.

Dress in loose fitting, layered clothing. You can remove a sweater or jacket if you feel the heat is too oppressive. Replace in moments.

Keep track of what seems to trigger hot flashes for you: anger, stress, spicy foods. Learn to minimize or avoid these provokers.

Stop smoking. Avoid excesive or all consumption of alcohol. Control your weight. Get plenty of rest.

Drink plenty of water. Eat fresh fruit or drink vegetable juices to help prevent urinary problems.

It has been suggested that red meats, caffeine, refined white sugars, and chocolate can all aggravate menopausal symptoms and perhaps should be avoided or kept to a minimum. Switch to a diet plentiful in fresh fruits and vegetables, whole grains, seafood, legumes, and low-fat dairy products.

Nutritional Therapy for Coping with the Change

Maintain a balance of calcium and phosphorous. Foods containing both these minerals include spinach, milk, and spaghetti. Having some of them throughout the week will help ease the reactions of the change.

You will also benefit from vitamins B-complex (found in whole grain foods), vitamin C (citrus fruits and juices), and vitamin D (in cod liver oil and from just a half-hour of sunshine a day). Your hormonal changes will be less noticeable if your body is fortified with these nutrients.

Vitamin E (whole grains and vegetable oils) are also helpful in easing the so-called transformation. *Caution:* People taking digitalis, a heart drug, should not take Vitamin E without a doctor's supervision.

You need more fiber or roughage. You will find this substance in bran, raw fruits, and vegetables and whole grain breads and cereals.

Exercise Is Important

At least 30 to 60 minutes a day is especially important. Activity helps your body to use calcium and other nutrients. Exercise strengthens the bones at a time of life when they are vulnerable to osteoporosis. *Tip:* Bicycling, walking, and swimming are three activities that are exceptionally important, do not strain the bones, and help you to cope with subtle hormonal changes.

The Vitamin That Soothes Menopausal Symptoms: Vitamin E

Vitamin E is considered a vasodilator in that it is able to open up constricted blood vessels and thereby permit a smooth flow throughout your circulatory system. During the menopause, you need to relieve congestion that may cause the "hot flushes" and related symptoms.

QUICK HELP FROM VITAMIN E

Upset by the recurring hot flushes, Anna G. decided to remedy the situation with the use of a simple vitamin program recommended by a local gynecologist. She took 200 units of vitamin E with each meal, for just three days. Then she reduced the dosage to just 200 per day with her noon meal. The symptoms just eased off, backed away, and rarely returned!

How Vitamins Help to Relieve Painful Problems

Among the classic problems presented by menopause for many women are leg cramps at night, frequent bruises, and nosebleed. These symptoms could be traced to capillary weaknesses, that is, weaknesses in the walls of the capillaries, which are the tiniest of the blood vessels.

Problem: There is a weakness in the walls of the capillaries, or tiniest of blood vessels. Pain may be caused by a shortage of oxygen in the muscles, because of poor functioning of the capillaries supplying those muscles. There is a high susceptibility to bruising because of thin-textured skin, defective cushioning of the deep vascular bed. A malnourished capillary system can cause nosebleed and other disorders.

Nutritional Therapy: You need to reinforce capillary resistance to stress and injury. You do so with vitamin C and the valuable bioflavonoids such as hesperidin and rutin. All are found in fresh fruits and their juices. In particular, the white netting under the peel of citrus fruits offers a therapeutic supply of the valuable nutrients. As stated earlier, be sure to have enough vitamin E, which keeps oxygen in the blood longer, an essential to treating such symptoms as leg cramps, hot flushes, headaches, irritability.

Just boost your intake of these citrus fruits and consider a supplement as recommended by your health practitioner. Menopause is a perfectly natural process. It should cause no more difficulty than any other basic bodily function. The key is, of course, a healthy body to begin with. The time to prepare for menopause is long, long before it arrives. And even after it has occurred, nutritional therapy will help you to cope with the change, without many changes.

IN A NUTSHELL

1. Menstrual difficulties are traced to a hormonal upheaval that can be controlled and eased with understanding and nutritional therapy.
2. Ease pain with such nutrients as vitamin B_6, calcium, zinc, potassium, vitamin E, tryptophan, and essential fatty acids, from foods as well as supplements.
3. To ease PMS distress, avoid salt, sugar, caffeine, but be sure to apply warmth to the painful area for soothing relief. Remember to exercise at least 30 to 60 minutes a day. Try the Comfort Pose if discomfort is severe. Spasms ease in minutes.
4. Carol DiG. overcame her disorders with a simple nutritional program with emphasis on items listed in this chapter.

5. As natural analgesics or pain relievers, try Muscle Relaxant Tonic, Mood Improvement Mix, Midday Pickup. They soothe spasms and make you feel happy. They're all natural, too!

6. Viola J. bid PMS "goodbye" with these natural pain relievers.

7. Be prepared for menopause or the big change of life. Cool off hot flashes with an improved picture of general health.

8. A group of specific vitamins are able to help take the flame out of the hot flashes of menopause.

9. Anna G. was able to relieve her disorders with a simple daily vitamin.

10. Use bioflavonoids to strengthen your capillaries and relieve leg cramps or ease bruising, which is all too unnecessarily common in menopause.

16

How Soothing Foods "Turn Off" Irritable Bowel Syndrome

Listen to your tummy talk. Those angry symptoms are trying to tell you something. A form of protest because of abuse or neglect or both. It is estimated that at least one out of every two tummy complaints center around irritable bowel syndrome (IBS).

In brief, you have cramps and alternating diarrhea and constipation, while nothing is wrong with your intestines. IBS is a name for a group of disorders in which various parts of the intestinal tract are inflamed The most common disorders are ulcerative colitis and Crohn's disease. Symptoms usually appear by age 25, are twice as common in women as in men, and may occur on and off for years.

Typical IBS Symptoms

A disturbed state of intestinal contractions for which no anatomical cause can be found. You may feel crampy abdominal pain, often with accompanying gasiness, diarrhea, or constipation, but a diagnostic search fails to show up any anatomic deformities. The problem is an essential disordered motility, that is, an upset in the muscular contractions of the intestines.

Stress Is a Clue to Intestinal Misbehavior

Your IBS could very well be stress related. Intestinal muscles tighten up and contract into spasm when you are emotionally upset. You are not alone. Virtually everybody responds to the stresses of life—anxiety, anger, frustration, depression—with some form of physical reaction. No part of the body is more vulnerable to these psychological disturbances than the gastrointestinal tract. The brain is "connected" to the muscles of this tract by a network of nerves. When you are emotionally upset, you can actually feel intestinal muscles tighten up and contract in spasms. Some people get headaches when under stress; others get vomiting spells, diarrhea, duodenal ulcers, and so on. All age groups are affected. For example, students and athletes often have nausea or diarrhea before an exam or sports event.

Eliminate "Food Triggers"

In addition to psychic factors, many substances can irritate the colon and trigger symptoms. You may respond if you eliminate "food triggers," which often include wheat, corn, sugar, spicy foods, coffee, tea, and alcohol; for some, dairy is irritating. You may have a lactose intolerance factor in which you find it upsetting to drink milk. If you notice such symptoms, you could eliminate these upsetting items. Many are relieved of IBS by cutting down on sugar, especially soda, pastries, and candy.

How Fiber Helps to Calm Your Irritated Bowels

The fiber of bulk foods (whole grains, raw vegetables, bran, wheat germ, for example) help to improve the motility of your colon. Fiber also lessens both the severity and frequency of IBS symptoms, which include crampy abdominal pain, constipation and/or diarrhea, and increased mucus, sometimes, in the stool. Dietary fiber substances found in coarse bran appear to reduce some of the pressures on the colon. This relaxes the colon, allowing normal transit to be restored, relieving IBS symptoms.

The ability of fiber to absorb and hold large volumes of water is an important benefit. For example, when bran absorbs the water, it swells and forms a mucilaginous gel. This promotes intestinal bulking and relief of cramps and irregularity. Fiber is an easy and effective form of nutritional therapy for IBS and related disorders.

Are You Fuzzy About Fiber?

Let's clear it up. Fiber is that rigid skeletal or cell wall portion of plant foods that slides through the small intestine without being digested. When it reaches the colon, it becomes fermented, but in that process, its bulk absorbs water and speeds elimination. Fiber has no nutrient allure. Its chief purpose is to form bulk, stabilize the bowel system, and ease distress. *Problem:* Without adequate fiber, the digestive process may slow down and constipation can develop, which in turn can lead to irritable bowel syndrome and related colonic upset.

The answer would be to increase fiber intake to help boost the health of your gastrointestinal system.

Easy Ways to Boost Fiber Consumption

Grandma called it roughage. She cautioned the family to eat whole grains, cereals, fruits, and vegetables. Her theories may have been scorned, but now they are revived and vindicated. What she called roughage, we now know as "fiber"—the key to healing and soothing irritable bowel syndrome, among other benefits. How can you "think fiber" for digestive happiness? One easy method is to use bran (the outer coating of seeds and grains).

Nutritional Therapy

Eat 1 or 2 tablespoons of bran each morning with your cereal and gradually build up to about ½ cup a day. Also, you could substitute whole grain breads such as rye or pumpernickle for white bread or rolls. Use brown (not white) rice. When you eat fresh fruits, eat the skins, too. Whenever edible, eat the skins of vegetables such as potatoes.

Simple Techniques

You can easily turn low-fiber foods into high-fiber foods. For example, whenever a recipe calls for bread crumbs, substitute bran. This works well with meatloaf or as a topping on tuna casserole. Noodle dishes can be made with whole wheat noodles. For dessert, try some granola sprinkled on yogurt. With a little imagination, you can think of many ways to get good taste into a high-fiber diet.

An easy rule of thumb is to include at least one serving of bran or whole grain in every meal—this could be cereal, bread, muffins, crackers, or brown rice. You should try to eat at least three servings of raw vegetables or fresh fruit every day.

How to Sneak Soothing Fiber into the Family Diet

- Buy baked goods and mixes made at least partly with whole grains (wheat, oats, rye, barley, corn) rather than just all-purpose flour.

- Add wheat germ, wheat bran, oat bran, All-bran cereal, or oatmeal to meat loaves and chilies. Substitute them for a small part of all-purpose flour in breads, muffins, or rolls.

- Toss cooked dried beans into soups and stews; garnish salads with them, too.

- At least twice a week, serve an all-vegetable meal.

- Snack on a handful of dry whole grain breakfast cereal, whole grain crackers, or popcorn rather than potato chips or pretzels.

- Serve brown rice or buckwheat groats (kasha) instead of white rice; serve whole wheat pasta instead of regular.

- Garnish salads with a sprinkle of nuts; or use spoon-sized shredded wheat as croutons.

- Substitute raisins, chopped figs, dates, or prunes in recipes calling for chocolate chips.

- At breakfast, in desserts, or when baking, concentrate on those fruits highest in fiber—bananas, apples, pears, raisins, prunes, and blueberries.

- Don't peel fruits and vegetables. Eat them with the skin on if you can.

- Eat corn, bran, or whole wheat muffins rather than doughnuts or pastry made with white flour.

You can actually eat your way to a healthier gastrointestinal system with the use of tasty fiber foods.

"HOPELESS" IBS BECOMES "HEALED" IN FOUR DAYS

Since his adolescence, William H. was troubled with colonic upset, diagnosed as IBS. He was told to live with the "hopeless" condition. His recurring abdominal pain, altered bowel habits, and constipation alternating with diarrhea was not life-threatening, but he often felt it was! Medications gave him temporary relief. But symptoms returned when they wore off. Prolonged use of harsh chemical laxatives led to dependency or just plain addiction! William H. feared his bowel could lose ability to function normally. He did not want to live with IBS. But he didn't know he could live without it.

A gastroenterologist recommended a fiber-boosting program as a means of forming bulk or roughage; the cellulose, hemicellulose, lignin, pectin, gums, and mucilages would absorb water and promote a normal movement, without the buildup of pressure resulting from strain.

William H. made this easy dietary change. He had more beans, whole grains, raw fruit, and vegetable salads and just 2 tablespoons of bran with his morning cereal, every single day. Within two days, cramps ended. Regularity was restored almost immediately. By the end of the fourth day, he no longer felt the abdominal pain and colonic distress. Fiber had "healed" his formerly "hopeless" IBS. He was free of this misdiagnosed lifetime affliction, thanks to daily intake of soothing fiber.

Five Steps to Better Health of the GI System

Improve the vigor and motility of your gastrointestinal system with these basic steps that restore youthful health to the colonic area:

1. Eat at regular hours, chewing your foods slowly and thoroughly.
2. Drink plenty of liquids, including fruit and vegetable juices, and water. Sufficient liquid intake is important to the function of the entire body, as well as that of the digestive tract.
3. Exercise daily. Take brisk walks, bicycle, jog, swim, or engage in any other sport you enjoy.
4. Be sensitive to your bowel function. Answer the "urge" for a movement promptly. If you delay, you may lose the urge and have to strain later on.
5. Avoid straining, if at all possible. Let nature take its course because too much straining can cause unnecessary irritation and even lead to hemorrhoids.

Tonics That Tame the Outraged Gastrointestinal System

How to cool off your inflamed colonic area? It is easy to reach for a chemical "fizz" tablet or powder. But the GI system becomes insensitive to repeated abuse and fails to work properly. Instead, tame and cool your flare-up with some soothing health tonics. They work in minutes. Relief spreads throughout your entire body and you sigh with contentment. They're refreshingly tasty, too.

Orange Fizz

Blenderize 1 peeled orange with 1 handful of nuts, 1 banana, 1 teaspoon of bran for just 2 minutes or until thoroughly combined. Now add to 8 ounces of plain, salt-free club soda. Stir vigorously. Drink this Orange Fizz whenever your IBS acts up. Within moments, the vitamins and minerals join with the fiber to coat your inflamed colon and provide a balm of contented relief. The fire is extinguished. The rumbling stops. What a wonderful feeling!

Morning Emulsion

Into a glass of sugar-free pineapple juice, add 1 teaspoon bran, 1 handful of sun-dried raisins, 1 scoop of plain yogurt. Blenderize for 3 minutes. Add to a glass of salt-free club soda. Stir vigorously. Drink this nose-tickling bubbly in the morning. Within moments, the bromelain enzymes of the pineapple juice join with the cellulose elements of the fiber and are both activated by the fructose of the raisins and propelled by the fermented elements of the yogurt. These substances gently but quickly break up the blockages in your GI System. The fizz bubbles of the club soda further disperse the congestion. In moments, this Morning Emulsion facilitates a smooth propelling of wastes to cool off inflammation and promote a natural elimination.

Quick Calm Cocktail

Combine 4 ounces of fat-free milk with 1 tablespoon bran, ½ cup of citrus fruits sections, and seasonal berries (raspberries and blackberries are tops in fiber). Blenderize for 2 minutes. Add to a ½ glass of salt-free club soda for enjoyment and palatability. Just sip slowly whenever you feel your tummy crying out with cramping rage. The calcium of the milk combines with the ascorbic acid of the fruit and the grain fiber along with the berry roughage to give you a feeling of emotional tranquility. Since much IBS can be traced to stress, just reach for the Quick Calm Cocktail and calm down those flurries. Within 15 minutes, you feel yourself relaxing all over, including your GI system.

Home Helps for Correction
of Constipation

A by-product of irritable bowel syndrome may often be constipation. It is a symptom, not a disease. Instead of relying upon harsh laxatives, eat a well-balanced diet that includes unprocessed bran, whole wheat bread, prunes and prune juices, and figs and fig juices. To stimulate activity, drink plenty of fluids and exercise regularly.

Apple + Water = Fast Relief

If you are bothered by difficulties in passing wastes, try this simple but amazingly swift-acting home remedy. Before breakfast, just eat two freshly washed and cored apples, skin and all. Follow with one or two glasses of freshly drawn water. (*No* ice water since it shocks and hurts your system.) Within moments, the fiber and pectin of the apple combine with the water to dislodge blockages and permit comfortable removal. Now you are ready for your high-fiber breakfast so you are protected against constipation in the near future.

FREES HERSELF FROM IRREGULARITY IN ONE DAY

Denise F. felt repeated cramps, bloating, and embarrassing constipation. This was part of the irritable bowel syndrome and overlapping irregularity. She tried laxatives, but they lost effectiveness and made her feel worse than before. Was there a natural remedy? Denise F. received the apple-plus-water before breakfast solution from a local homeopathic physician. She tried it. Miraculously, within one day, the IBS and constipation just "went away." By continuing this simple prebreakfast remedy, she never again had constipation. The IBS symptoms just faded away. A simple but effective nutritional therapy!

Nutritional Therapy for Irregularity

Boost roughage intake with such foods as whole grains, bran, cabbage, cauliflower, asparagus, tomatoes, onions, and legumes. Fruits such as apples, pears, oranges, grapes, figs, raisins, and prunes are also helpful. Honey, too, has a mildly laxative effect. A glass of hot water with the juice of a ½ lemon and 1 teaspoon of honey, taken on arising, is beneficial. *Tip:* Prunes contain *isatin,* apparently a laxative factor. A handful of pitted prunes or a glass of prune juice in the morning on an empty stomach may be all you need to get back on the regular track.

Are You Milk Intolerant?

The inability to digest milk and milk products properly may be due to your deficiency of lactase, the intestinal enzyme that digests the sugar found in milk. The symptoms, which include cramps, gas, bloating, and diarrhea, appear 15 minutes to several hours after consuming milk or a milk product.

You may manage the problem by eating fewer dairy products, taking smaller servings more frequently, or adding a special nonprescription preparation to milk that makes it easier to digest. It is available in health stores and pharmacies.

Try fermented dairy products—yogurt, buttermilk, cheese—because the lactose has been partially predigested. Also try these low-lactose cheeses: brick, uncreamed cottage cheese, Brie, Camembert, cheddar, Edam, Gouda, Limburger, provolone, and Stilton. *Tip:* Milk-containing foods are better tolerated if in a *warm* form than if very cold. You may not experience symptoms if you drink a glass of comfortably *hot* milk, in small sips.

If fewer dairy foods are eaten, other products that have calcium (such as dark green leafy vegetables, salmon, and bean curd) should be substituted to help keep the bones strong.

With soothing foods, you can strengthen your gastrointestinal region to help "turn off" any irritation so that you enjoy a healthy and contented digestive system!

MAIN POINTS

1. Irritable bowel syndrome may be traced to emotional upset. If you control stress, you resist intestinal outrage.

2. Be cautious of "food triggers" that can cause digestive explosions.

3. Fiber is able to calm your irritated bowels. Use this simple substance to help correct IBS.

4. Sneak soothing fiber into the family diet with the tasteful suggestions for all meal occasions.

5. William H. was healed of "hopeless" IBS in four days on an easy high-fiber program of nutritional therapy.

6. Just five simple steps help you enjoy improved health of your gastrointestinal system.

7. Tame stomach outrage with the refreshing health tonics made in minutes. They work just as swiftly.

8. Denise F. freed herself from irregularity with a simple apple-water remedy in the morning.

9. Lactose intolerance can be eased with simple dietary adjustments.

17

Enrich Your Bloodstream for a Youthful Body and Mind

When it comes to rejuvenation, iron is a metal more precious than gold. Iron is the mineral that enriches your bloodstream, builds immunity to premature aging, regulates your body temperature, and even affects your ability to learn and concentrate. Iron is a "whole body" nutrient that gives you a youthful body and mind. Iron-packed red blood cells carry energy-giving oxygen to every part of your body. The key to total rejuvenation lies in an enriched bloodstream.

Iron Builds Immunity

Phagocytes (white blood cells that serve as your body's primary defense mechanism against bacterial infections) depend on iron-containing enzymes to do their immune building. These cells engulf bacteria and release corrosive substances, such as oxidants, that digest the invading microbe once it is engulfed. Phagocytes need much oxygen to produce detoxifying substances. It is iron in your bloodstream that brings them the breath of life.

Iron Resists Infections

Lymphocytes (immune-building and infection-fighting white blood cells) produce antibodies to ward off the risk of infection. These cells need iron for energy metabolism and for the production of enzymes vital to their specialized roles in the immune response. The production of antibodies also requires iron-dependent enzymes.

Iron Fights Viruses

Most viral diseases, including genital herpes, may become worse with iron-deficient blood. The reason is that lymphocytes, the major defense against viral infections, also need iron for optimal activity. To help resist a viral infection, your blood must be enriched with valuable iron stores.

Iron Improves Intelligence

Iron helps your brain release chemicals called catecholamines that are involved in the function of the central nervous system. Iron-containing enzymes create a balance of neurotransmitters to improve behavior and learning abilities. With iron-produced brain chemicals, there is a significant improvement in attention span and cooperativeness. You learn better. Your brain seems able to "receive" more information because of this iron-improved condition.

With a healthy bloodstream, you have hopes for a younger body and mind—at any age!

How to Wake Up Your "Tired Blood"

If you are troubled with cold hands and feet, constant chills, a pale complexion, lowered resistance to infection, and a breakdown in your immune system, you may have an iron deficiency. This mineral is needed to make hemoglobin, the pigment in red blood cells that carries energy-producing oxygen to your millions of tissues from head to toe.

A deficiency of iron intake or absorption results in a reduced hemoglobin supply with such telltale symptoms as chronic fatigue, lassitude, pallid skin, malformed nails, pale mucous membranes, shortages of breath, headache, and emotional weakness.

In short, you have "tired blood." To nourish your hemoglobin, feed it iron and wake up your body and mind with new youth.

Risks of an Iron Deficiency

Iron is stored in your bone marrow, liver, and spleen. When your body does not get enough iron, you will begin to deplete these stores. At this point, you may look and feel fine, but a shock to your system, such as a cold or flu or dieting, can cause you to become anemic.

Energy Level Impaired

This is a condition in which there is a reduction in the amount and size of the red blood corpuscles or in the amount of hemoglobin, or both. When you become anemic, your body's ability to carry oxygen may actually be reduced to 75 percent of its normal oxygen-carrying capability. When less oxygen reaches your muscles, it can reduce the amount of energy that can be produced, leaving you pale, weakened, and tired. In more advanced conditions, there is poor appetite, gastrointestinal disturbances, difficult breathing.

Immune System Impaired

Insufficient iron can also reduce your body's resistance to bacteria and illness. Your body's immune system depends on iron-containing enzymes and sufficient oxygen to function properly.

How Much Iron Do You Need?

The adult body contains about 3 to 4 grams of iron, which is slowly absorbed from food in the small intestine and passes in the blood to the bone marrow. Here it is used to manufacture red blood cells. A basic rule of thumb is to obtain 10 milligrams daily for men and 18 milligrams daily for women. *Special needs:* A minimum of 18 milligrams daily is necessary for adolescent girls and women throughout their reproductive years because of menstruation and child-bearing demands. Adolescent boys should receive 18 milligrams of iron daily because of rapid growth. *Important:* Dieters, because of the lower calorie intake, are at high risk of iron-deficient blood. Very active women make up still another high-risk group. Increased physical activity can cause greater red cell destruction that, in turn, increases your need for iron.

Easy Ways to "Ironize" Your Bloodstream

Enrich your rivers of life through nutritional therapy with your knife and fork. Some tasty iron-enrichment methods include the following along with those listed in Chart 17-1.

1. Liver is a rich source of iron. It also has a considerable fat and cholesterol, so use smaller portions, just once a week.
2. Dried beans and peas (cholesterol-free) are great sources of iron as well as protein. Both combine to improve blood health.
3. Lima beans, green peas, and dark green leafy vegetables such as kale, collards, and turnip greens are great sources of iron from a meatless source. Feature them often.

4. Sun-dried fruits used as a snack, as a dessert, or mixed in with your cereal will increase iron in your bloodstream.

5. Enriched or whole grain flour, breads, cereals, rolls, corn meal, macaroni, spaghetti, and noodles will give you top sources of iron as well as appreciable protein.

6. Cook and bake in cast iron pots. This will help put more iron into the food.

Chart 17-1: FOODS THAT SUPPLY IRON

Food	Serving Size	Milligrams of Iron
Bread Group		
Wheat bran	⅓ cup	4.9
Yeast, brewer's	3 tbsp.	4.0
Soybeans, cooked	⅓ cup	1.8
Beans, common, cooked	⅓ cup	1.8
Wheat germ	¼ cup	1.8
Bread, whole grain	1 slice	.5–.6
Milk Group		
Skim milk	8 ounces	.1
Vegetable Group		
Spinach, cooked	½ cup	2.0
Peas, green, cooked	½ cup	1.4
Brussels sprouts, cooked	6 to 7	1.1
Chard, cooked	⅗ cup	1.8
Fruit Juice		
Prune juice	¼ cup	2.5
Strawberries, raw	1 cup	1.5
Meat Group		
Liver	1 ounce	2.6
Turkey or duck	1 ounce	1.7
Egg	1 medium	1.2
Beef, veal	1 ounce	1.0
Tofu	½ cup	1.7
Snacks		
Pumpkin seeds	2 tsp.	1.0

Vitamin C + Iron = Rich Bloodstream

Be sure to take any vitamin C food or beverage *together* with your iron food for better absorption and assimilation. *Example:* fruit slices or juice with a small portion of meat, fish, or poultry.

Vitamin C Sources

Citrus fruits are high in this nutrient. You may enjoy oranges, grapefruit, tomatoes, cantaloupes, strawberries, papayas, mangoes, guavas, raw cabbage, green pepper, broccoli, cauliflower, Brussels sprouts, potatoes, turnip greens, and kale. *Note:* Cooking tends to destroy vitamin C, so try to include as many raw foods as possible. (Try raw potato sticks, cut as thin as matchsticks.)

Common Iron Robbers and How to Avoid Them

Protect your iron reserves from "theft" by these reactions:

Commercial Tea, Coffee

The tannic acid and/or caffeine of these beverages bind to the iron in your meal and make it impossible to be absorbed. If you drink tea or coffee with your meal or shortly thereafter, you can decrease iron absorption by nearly 40 percent.

Food Additives

EDTA and phosphates, found in soft drinks and processed baked goods and other foods can inhibit iron absorption.

Excessive Fiber

High-fiber diets can also block iron absorption. It would be best to take an iron supplement *before* your fiber meal by at least several hours to avoid antagonism.

Antacids

They decrease the ability of gastric enzymes to dissolve dietary iron.

Industrial Pollutants

These common chemical fallouts such as cadmium and lead are also known iron inhibitors.

Stress, Tension

It can drain away your vitamin and mineral reserves, including iron!

Best Blood with Vitamin B$_{12}$

Also known as cobalamin, this vitamin is needed for a rich bloodstream. But it does much more. A deficiency of vitamin B$_{12}$ leads to nerve tissue deterioration, sore back, numbness and tingling in the feet, diminished vibration sense, along with emotional and nervous weaknesses.

Vitamin B$_{12}$ enriches your bloodstream and then enriches your total body health. Your needs are small, at least 3 micrograms daily. To obtain it, you need to have skim milk, eggs (again, high in cholesterol so use in moderation), cheddar cheese, seafood, and liver.

Missing in Meatless Foods

Because vitamin B$_{12}$ does not occur in plant products, you would need to take a supplement if you are on a meatless diet.

A well-nourished bloodstream is your key to a healthy and vigorous mind and body.

FEELS "RESTORED TO LIFE" WITH NOURISHED BLOODSTREAM

Susan B. would huddle under several sweaters even in the warmest of weather. She had a rapid heartbeat upon the slightest of exertion. Her skin was becoming thick and dry, losing its youthful stretchability. The linings of her mouth and eyes turned from a healthy pink to a pale or sallow color. She complained of nervousness, headache, and loss of appetite. She felt she was aging rapidly. She was not even 50 years of age!

During an examination, her internist observed her constant shivering and listened to her complaints of tiredness and feeling "just plain old." He diagnosed her condition as malnourished blood. He told Susan B. to boost her intake of iron-rich foods such as liver (small portion, once a week); prune juice; beans; whole grain iron-fortified, and sugar-free, salt-free cereals; sunflower seed kernels; and seafoods. She was to avoid coffee and tea (except caffeine-free and

218

tannin-free) and food additives. This simple nutritional therapy would give her bloodstream the needed nutrients to provide vigor to her system.

Susan B. followed the simple and tasty iron-enriched program. Within five days, she felt much younger. She no longer had to overdress. Her heartbeat was pronounced healthy. Her skin glowed. She was calm and alert and had a healthy appetite.

Nutritional therapy aimed at enriching the bloodstream had made her look "too young"; she laughed as she said she was glad to be "restored to life."

How To Cook Up an Iron Supply

Cast iron cookware boosts iron content of the food. For example, when acid foods such as tomatoes are prepared in iron cookware, varying amounts of organic iron are formed.

In some cases, food cooked in iron cookware can have three to four times more iron than can the same foods cooked in glass or stainless steel. Spaghetti sauce, for example, cooked for about 20 minutes in an iron pot contains 6 milligrams of iron per 3½ ounces. But iron levels in that same amount of sauce prepared in a glass pot amount to only 3 milligrams. The iron content of scrambled eggs, brown rice casserole, and gravy more than doubles when cooked in an iron pot. *Tip:* You could cook in an iron wok and boost your mineral reserves without much effort.

Caution: Iron can be water soluble. Use a cooking method that minimizes losses. Steam or cook vegetables in small amounts of water, for the shortest possible time. Be sure to use vegetable stocks for soups, casseroles, and gravies.

You can cook yourself a blood-enriching supply of iron in these tasty methods.

Sample Menu High in Food Iron

Try this iron- and vitamin-rich menu plan to help nourish your bloodstream and body.

Breakfast: ½ grapefruit; ⅔ cup cream of wheat; 1 slice wholegrain toast; 1 pat margarine; 1 cup milk, fruit juice.

Lunch: Tuna salad sandwich with 2 slices whole grain bread, 3 ounces tuna salad, lettuce, and tomato; 1 medium apple; 4 medium carrot sticks; fruit or vegetable juice.

Dinner: 3 ounces broiled ground beef patty; 1 cup baked beans; mixed green salad with 1 tablespoon dressing; ½ cup fruit cocktail without sugar; 1 cup milk.

Snack: 2 tablespoons peanut butter with salt-free crackers.

Your Iron Intake: A whopping 25 milligrams!

SIMPLE DIET CHANGE RESCUES MAN FROM ANEMIA

A blood test showed that salesman Jon O'N. was running the risk of anemia. This condition is said to exist if the hemoglobin level falls more than 2 grams below "normal." In males, 14 to 16 grams of hemoglobin per 100 cubic centimeters of blood is considered normal; in women, 12 to 14 grams is normal. Jon's tests showed a drop in his hemoglobin, to below 10 grams.

He looked pale and wan. He was so cranky, he snapped at company supervisors and, worse, potential as well as existing customers. His sales chart showed a downward slide. He had such a pasty complexion, he would "turn off" persons in authority.

His supervisor insisted he be examined by a hematologist or blood specialist. He had recognized the same "tired blood" symptoms in his wife and seen her bounce back to good health with a diet correction. Jon O'N. was examined and told to boost iron intake on a simple diet change. Daily, include several items from the accompanying list of iron-containing foods. Follow the menu plan, too. Results? In just six days, he was cheerful, glowed with the picture of a healthy youth and had so much energy, he soon had a sales record that "went through the ceiling" thanks to his revived bloodstream!

Garlic: The Food Your Blood Must Have

Garlic is known for having antihemolytic factors; namely, it is able to promote the increase of red cells and hemoglobin in the bloodstream and give your rivers of life a supercharging of vitality and energy.

Garlic is also rich in allicin, a substance that protects against bacterial infection and other blood disorders. Garlic also contains alliin (a sulfur-containing amino acid) which has an antibiotic effect to "knock out" and "defuse" the proliferation of potentially harmful wastes floating in your bloodstream. *No other food has this amazing blood-building power!*

For a richer and healthier bloodstream, be sure to have several garlic cloves daily.

220

How to Take Garlic

Use a few cloves in cooked soups, stews, casseroles, baked vegetables, and meat dishes. Dice a clove or two and add to your vegetable salad. Use diced garlic for sandwich spreads. Blenderize several vegetables with a few garlic cloves for a tangy and refreshing blood-nourishing drink.

Iron Tonic to Wake Up Your "Tired Blood"

Blenderize 1 tablespoon of wheat bran, 2 tablespoons brewer's yeast, ½ cup salt-free tomato juice, ½ cup skim milk, ¼ cup prune juice, and 2 garlic cloves. Whiz until thoroughly combined.

Drink this Iron Tonic in the morning, preferably before breakfast. The rich iron combines with the garlic and the other vitamins and minerals to sweep away the cobwebs from your bloodstream and give you a wide-awake look and feel physically and mentally. It works in minutes! It lasts for days!

LOOK YOUNGER, FEEL ALERT IN MINUTES

Marcia L. not only looked pale and felt lackadaisical, her vital signs were always sluggish. She felt old beyond her 40 years. Her breathing difficulties and lack of resistance to colds made her look and act like an invalid!

A nutritionist diagnosed the condition as impoverished blood. Marcia L. was told to boost iron-containing foods and cooking methods. At the same time, she was told to drink the Iron Tonic every morning until she felt well. In just one day, the tonic worked like a miracle! She had roses in her cheeks, was filled with energy, breathed normally, and had youthful resistance against infectious bacteria. Thanks to the Iron Tonic (she drinks it daily to guard against "tired blood"), she was restored to youth, in minutes!

Your body's vital fluid can be "revived" with the use of iron and other essential nutrients. It may be needed in small quantities, but without enough of a supply, it could cause a deficiency that may very well age your body and mind. Had your iron today?

IN REVIEW

1. Iron is a trace element that builds immunity, resists infections, fights viruses, and improves intelligence.

2. Note the list of six easy ways to "ironize" your bloodstream.

3. Vitamin C plus iron consumed at the same time is the key to a rich bloodstream.

4. Protect against "iron theft" by little-known threats to your blood health.

5. Build a richer bloodstream with vitamin B_{12}.

6. Susan B. was "restored to life" on an iron-enrichment program.

7. Plan your daily meal program with the use of any of the iron-containing foods.

8. You can use certain cooking methods to double and triple iron supply of ordinary foods.

9. Jon O'N. overcame anemia and ill health on a simple diet change.

10. Garlic is a "must" food for blood health.

11. Marcia L. was able instantly to "ironize" her blood with the use of a tangy and revitalizing Iron Tonic.

──18──

Healing Your Vital Organs with Nutritional Therapy

Y our midsection organs may have an occasional upset or repeated difficulties crying out for help. Symptoms are your vital organs' way of signaling how they are working. Learning to read messages sent by your organs is important, both for self-care and for knowing when to seek professional help. Let us take a closer look at several of your most important vital organs and see how to answer any calls of trouble with nutritional therapy. Better still, we shall see how to revitalize your organs so they are in youthful health and remain free of disturbance.

Your Gallbladder

Your gallbladder is a pear-shaped sac located beneath the liver on the right-hand side of the abdominal cavity. Its primary job is to collect and store bile, a cholesterol-rich digestive juice secreted by the liver and pumped into the small intestine each time you eat. When digestion is completed, the bile is routed to the gallbladder for storage.

Bile breaks up fat so that it can be further digested by pancreatic enzymes and absorbed by the intestines. Bile contains bile salts, cholesterol, bilirubin (bile pigment formed from hemoglobin when red blood cells are broken down), and lecithin (a waxy substance capable of dissolving fats). In one day, as much as 700 milliliters (almost 3 cups) of bile aid in digestion.

When Problems Happen

In many people, bile becomes so saturated with cholesterol that it can no longer remain in solution. That is, it is no longer liquid and free moving. It forms crystal particles that slowly develop into stones. *Symptoms:* There could be a sudden intense pain in the upper right side of the abdomen that builds to a peak over a few hours, then fades as the

223

stone is either passed out with the bile or falls back into the gallbladder where it becomes stuck in the bile duct.

Who Gets Gallstones?

More susceptible are women who have been pregnant; also at risk are overweight people who eat excessive amounts of animal fats and folks over age 60. Basically, those who are "female, fat, and forty" are most likely to develop gallstones.

Nutritional Therapy

To strengthen your resistance against gallbladder distress, certain food groups can have a therapeutic benefit. These include the following:

1. *Boost fiber intake.* Whether from whole grains or raw fruits and vegetables or legumes, fiber is important to protect against an excess production of a substance called deoxycholic acid, a substance that encourages gallstone formation. Fiber keeps this deoxycholic acid under control to protect against overload and risk of crystallization of bile.

2. *Low animal fat diet.* Cholesterol-containing foods are linked to gallbladder disease. If you consume a fatty meal, the bile becomes "saturated" with cholesterol. This excess calcifies into rock hard stones. Reduce intake of animal fatty foods, and you reduce fatty overload and the risk of stone formation.

3. *Increase complex carbohydrate foods.* They help to clear more cholesterol from your gallbladders to protect against their isolation and formation into stones. Such cholesterol-washing foods include raw fruits and vegetables and whole grains, particularly bran in your cereal or baked goods. *Suggestion:* Begin each meal with a large raw vegetable salad; end each meal with a raw fruit selection.

4. *Try soybeans for bladder health.* In particular, soy milk (available at health stores and special diet food outlets) is important for building gallbladder health. Soy milk is said to have a solubilizing effect on existing or threatening gallstones, helping to protect against enlargement and preparing the crystals for excretion. *Suggestion:* Use soy milk with your high-fiber bran and fruit cereal for speedy

washing out of accumulated crystals and protect against stone formation.

5. *Garlic is good for gallbladder.* Eaen daily, garlic has a detoxifying effect on the body, neutralizing the effect of saturated cholesterol, cleansing the bile, and enabling it to use lecithin to dissolve ingested fats. Garlic has important fat-dissolving properties to help keep your bladder "slim" and clean. In particular, garlic contains the potent diallyldisulphide-oxide. This compound has powerful cholesterol and fat-fighting effects that can uproot, dislodge, and wash out accumulated deposits that could otherwise shape into stones. *Suggestion:* With your raw salad, add two or three diced garlic cloves. Use in vegetable loaves and baked casseroles. Blenderize one chopped garlic clove in a glass of tomato juice and drink as a healthy tonic.

With these simple but effective dietary programs, you can reduce and even eliminate the risk of cholesterol-filled gallstones.

NUTRITION SAVES HOUSEWIFE FROM GALLSTONE SURGERY

Wanda LeG. was troubled with recurring pain, usually sudden, often severe, in the middle and right portions of her abdomen. At times, she perspired heavily and had a chill with a high fever. Her gastroenterologist said she was developing some gallstones, and from diagnostic tests, they could be serious. He told her she may have to undergo surgery and possible removal of the gallbladder.

She sought an alternative outlet. A second opinion from a weight specialist confirmed the presence of crystallized stones, but surgery was not imminent. Instead, the specialist used nutritional therapy. Wanda LeG. reduced animal fat intake, simultaneously increasing meatless foods and high complex carbohydrates. Daily, she would drink one glass of the tomato juice plus garlic tonic. She included fresh fruits, raw vegetables, and whole grains plus soy milk on a daily basis. Her weight dropped quickly. Within 19 days, the accumulated crystals had liquified and were washed out of her system. Her specialist confirmed that not were her symptoms gone, so were the threatening stones! She was saved from surgery, thanks to nutritional therapy.

You need not get stuck with gallstones! Fight back with the use of more meatless foods and home remedies and have a healthy gallbladder.

Your Kidneys

These are your body's filter plants, through which some 150 quarts of fluid pass every day. The fact that you have two kidneys gives you a wider margin of safety. If something should go wrong with one, you can get along satisfactorily with just the other. But your goal is to keep both of your kidneys in good health.

Each kidney is made up of a million tiny filters. These filters strain waste products (chiefly those left from protein digestion) out of the blood, dissolve them in water, and excrete them in the form of urine. The blood enters one end of each tiny tube in the kidney and is forced to leave through the other end, which is much smaller. All this adds up to a very effective filtering system.

If any of these units goes out of operation, the waste products in the blood cannot be thrown off and difficulties develop.

When Problems Happen

Foremost are kidney stones, or calcium oxalate urinary stones. These are primarily produced in the kidneys. If they are small enough, they could pass out of the body through the urinary tract, frequently causing excruciating discomfort in the process. Otherwise, they may obstruct the tube leading from the kidney and cause painful difficulties necessitating surgical removal. That is, the stones are removed, not the kidney.

Another problem is that of nephritis or Bright's disease. These are general terms used to describe the many forms of renal (kidney) disease that can cause inflammation. It may ultimately destroy the tiny membranes and microscopic filtering units, or nephrons, inside the kidneys. The damage caused by nephritis includes kidney failure and uremia; that is, toxic waste products accumulate to dangerous concentrations in the blood.

Nutritional Therapy

To help improve the health of your kidneys, institute a regeneration and cleansing program that will help to keep the filtering process in smooth function.

1. *Avoid destructive foods.* Salt, pepper, and alcohol (if these can be properly called foods!) should be restricted or totally eliminated.

They are kidney irritants that pass through these vital organs and can erode the delicate tissues and tubules. Often, a simple elimination will help to protect against stone formation and cool off the inflammation of Bright's disease.

2. *Avoid chemicalized analgesics.* You know them as pain killers or aspirin. These drug compounds usually contain phenacetin or acetominophen which are irritating to the kidneys. In some reported situations, excessive or habitual use of such drugs was directly responsible for injury to the kidneys. Because kidney metabolism and its structure are extremely complex, the kidneys are ever in danger of injury from chemical compounds.

3. *Less animal fat, more fiber.* Kidney stones, being made mainly of calcium oxalate, can be resisted or avoided on a low-animal-fat program. The reason is that excessive meat (animal fat and protein) causes the urine to become oversaturated calcium oxalate, the very substance from which stones are made. Moreover, refined carbohydrates contribute to accumulation of calcium oxalate salts and stones. Yet, when dietary fiber, along with whole grain complex carbohydrates, are consumed, calcium absorption and excretion become normalized, reducing the risk of stone formation. (Vegetarians seem to have a lower incidence of kidney stone formation.) Fiber is unique in that it "sponges up" bile acid secretions and urinary calcium and oxalate excretions and then removes these kidney threats via eliminative channels.

4. *Drink lots of water daily.* From six to eight glasses daily may well be the best and safest treatment for your kidneys. Water can prevent stones by diluting bile acids and helping wash them out of the system. Water also keeps the calcium oxalate crystals from sticking together. Instead, water just swirls the specks around in your kidneys and prepares them to be cleansed from your system.

5. *Increase consumption of magnesium.* This trace element makes the urine more solvent in respect to oxalates. With greater solvency, the fluid holds the crystals in solution with less risk of precipitation or aggregation, that is, the clumping together of particles. Plan to include such magnesium-containing foods as brewer's yeast, wheat bran, wheat germ, and raw green, leafy vegetables in your daily meal plan. Your health practitioner can advise you on magnesium supplements.

6. *Be generous with vitamin B_6.* Also known as pyridoxine, it works with magnesium to help control the body's production of oxalic acid and therefore to limit the amount reaching the kidneys. Vitamin B_6 also helps to protect against nephritis (inflammation). It works *together* with magnesium in nourishing your kidneys and rebuilding the health of these organs. This *combination* effect means your daily program of nutritional therapy should include both of these nutrients. Vitamin B_6 is found in brewer's yeast, wheat bran, wheat germ, raw mushrooms, raw broccoli, and raw cauliflower; modest amounts are in oranges, strawberries, and squash.

7. *Sweat it out.* In some situations, in the early stages of kidney difficulties, a sweat bath or sauna (hot, dry heat) could be useful. When the kidneys are unable to flush sufficient wastes from the blood, these materials can build up to threaten health. An alternative route is for these wastes to be released through sweating. In particular, stored-up urea nitrogen can be washed out through your perspiration and reduce or even eliminate risk of uremia. *Caution:* Check with your health practitioner to determine your eligibility for taking sauna baths. Certain cardiovascular conditions preclude excessive heat of any sort.

With this easy seven-step nutritional and health therapy plan, you can help keep your kidneys in tip-top shape.

KIDNEY STONES JUST "GO AWAY" WITH CORRECTIVE NUTRITION

District salesman Ronald O'K. admitted neglecting healthy nutrition and the need for daily intake of liquids. This inattention to his own bodily needs brought on abdominal pains and inflammation that his internist diagnosed as kidney stoneprone! Fortunately, the internist was aware of nutritional therapy and recommended the preceding seven-step program, including approved "sweats." Within two weeks, Ronald O'K.'s pains and inflammation cooled off; a new diagnosis confirmed that the disorder had cleared up and the threat of kidney stones just seemed to "go away." And all this without any medication!

Kidney Correction Health Tonic

To 1 glass of orange juice, add 1 teaspoon of wheat germ, 1 teaspoon of brewer's yeast, and several strawberries. Whiz together for 2 minutes. Drink just 1 glass daily. Morning is best. The rich concentration of magnesium with the B_6 help to liquefy any crystals and wash them out of your system. This Kidney Correction Health Tonic also cools off that inflammation associated with sweating and discomfort. Works in minutes, too!

Your Liver

After the skin, your liver is the largest organ of your body. It is a master laboratory, filtering out undesirable substances, neutralizing waste materials, manufacturing organic compounds, and storing nutrients to be released into the bloodstream when your body needs them.

Your liver is located on the right side of your abdomen, a little below your waistline where it is part of your digestive system.

Your liver stores iron and fibrogen, two valuable parts of the blood. When needed to heal, these substances are speedily dispatched. This organ is very sensitive to all chemical and physical changes in the body. It cooperates with the kidneys, the gallbladder, and the pancreas to accomplish its work. Because it filters out poisons and wastes, it should be protected with your very life! Without a liver, there is *no* life!

When Problems Happen

Common disorders include viral hepatitis (meaning inflammation). Hepatitis A is spread through contaminated water and food. Hepatitis B is acquired from transfusions or other blood products. It can be transmitted through tiny cuts or abrasions or by such simple acts as kissing, tooth brushing, ear piercing, tattooing, having dental work, or during sexual contact. In hepatitis, the liver becomes tender and enlarged; symptoms include fever, weakness, nausea, jaundice, and aversion to food.

The second serious problem is cirrhosis of the liver, a degenerative disorder where liver cells are damaged and replaced by scar formation. As scar tissue progressively accumulates, blood flow through the liver is diminished, causing even more cells to die. The liver becomes tawny and characteristically knobby due to nodules.

Loss of liver function results in gastrointestinal disturbances, emaciation, enlargement of not only the liver but the spleen (located on the left side of the body below and behind the stomach to act as a blood reservoir), jaundice, and accumulation of fluid in the abdomen and other body tissues. Anything that results in severe liver injury can cause cirrhosis. About half of fatalities of cirrhosis are caused by alcohol abuse, hepatitis, and other viruses. Some chemicals, many poisons, and obstruction of the bile duct can also cause cirrhosis.

Nutritional Therapy

Your goal is to rebuild your midsection because all organs are so interconnected and interdependent. Zero in on your liver with nutrients and basic home remedies that revitalize this important organ and give you a feeling of youthful health.

1. *Avoid alcohol.* Alcohol cancels any benefits from nutrition. So you must stop drinking to improve your nutrition.

2. *Increase intake of choline.* A member of the B-complex vitamin family, it has been found to control liver lipids (fats) and nourish the cells. Choline helps to transform liver fats into phospholipids to maintain good health. Without them, there is a backup of accumulated fat droplets that form cystlike structures within the liver cells. Such an infiltration renders the liver helpless to detoxify poisons or metabolize nutrients. You will find choline in a food supplement, lecithin; it is also abundant in soybeans as well as egg yolk, which, unfortunately, has an abundance of cholesterol. Some choline is found in egg white, so use this freely because it is cholesterol-free. Choline is also available as a supplement.

3. *Increase intake of zinc.* This mineral contains an enzyme called "superoxide dismutase" which directly inhibits peroxidation or the formation of free radicals, harmful fragments that can break down liver health. Zinc tends to protect liver cells from toxins such as the industrial chemicals carbon tetrachloride, a dry cleaning solvent, and hydrazine, an ingredient in the making of jet fuel. Zinc is found in wheat germ, wheat bran, brown rice, blackeye peas, and nuts. Zinc is also available as a supplement.

4. *Control animal fat intake.* It tends to cling to the liver and cause overload of the tissues, sometimes blocking the free flow of movement of important nutrients. Too much fat storage in your liver is detrimental to your health. Opt for low-fat animal foods and more whole grains, legumes, and seafoods.

5. *Vitamin E to the rescue.* According to some reports, vitamin E can protect against liver injury when blood flow to that organ has been cut off. Vitamin E inhibits the production of peroxidized fats that

occurs with the return of blood flow. Those fats are responsible for liver injury. Vitamin E is found in whole grain breads, cereals, wheat germ, wheat bran, and many cold-pressed oils, as well as a supplement.

6. *Avoid salt.* It triggers the kidneys to remove too much water from the system, irritating the liver and causing forms of erosion to the delicate tubules, especially the area involved with cirrhosis. Excess salt could give rise to *ascites,* meaning an accumulation of fluid in the abdomen. You will have a healthier liver and one that can be regenerated more speedily on a salt-free program.

7. *Remember your vitamin C.* You need to establish healthy metabolism to protect against liver injury. To make sure your liver keeps regulating your metabolism to a healthy degree, keep it nourished with enough vitamin C. This is a known fighter of toxic substances. It improves resistance of the liver to antagonistic toxins. This nutrient is found in fresh citrus fruits and juices, many vegetables, as well as in supplement.

RECOVERS FROM LIVER INJURY ON EASY NUTRITIONAL THERAPY

Concerned when her skin turned sallow and she felt feverish and weak, Dolores S. was examined by an internist who said her liver needed nutritional help. He suggested the preceding seven-step program. Nothing else. In six days, her condition improved. Dolores S. had youthful skin, was no longer feverish, and had bouncy energy, thanks to a rejuvenated liver via nutritional therapy!

Garlic Breathes New Life into Polluted Liver

Your liver is constantly threatened by heavy-metal poisoning! Lead, mercury, cadmium, arsenic, and copper come from polluted air, not to mention industrial and other sources. Copper enters the body from commonly used copper water pipes. This presents a constant threat to the health of the liver as well as the body.

Remember, everything filters through your liver, including pollutants! Over a period of time, you may develop toxic effects from heavy-metal poisoning.

You need not just sit there and take it. Fight back with garlic! This tangy vegetable is able to protect against the poisoning effect of heavy metals and cleanse your erythrocyte membrane from disintegration.

Garlic seems to attach itself to lead, mercury, and cadmium and prepares them for elimination. Otherwise, they might be stored in your liver to cause inner erosion.

By eating several cloves of garlic a day, you will help to neutralize and detoxify your liver and remove the threat of inner pollution. Whether diced in salads or added to cooked meals, garlic may well be the most effective nutritional therapy your vital organs need to keep you alive and well and youthful!

Begin youthful health in the middle…of your body! Keep your vital gallbladder, kidney, and liver in top-notch health, and the rest of your body and mind will share in that look and feel of total youth.

HIGHLIGHTS

1. Be good to your gallbladder with the five-step nutritional therapy program.
2. Wanda LeG. saved herself from gallstone surgery with this simple and effective food program.
3. Treat your kidneys with kindness by nourishing them with the seven-step better health program.
4. Corrective nutrition helped Ronald O'K. who was troubled with the threat of kidney stones. They seemed to just "go away" on the seven-step prescribed program.
5. Soothe your liver with loving nutritional care. A seven-step program helps it enjoy a new lease on life.
6. Dolores S. used this program to recover from liver injury.
7. Remember to include garlic on a daily basis as a shield and healer for your polluted liver.

How Foods Can Strengthen Your Life Saving Immune System

Nutritional therapy, working at the cellular level, can strengthen your resistance to almost any threat ranging from the common cold to the high risk of cancer. Specific food groups are able to help your body win the battle against invasion by microorganisms, be they bacteria or viruses. These foods are able to rebuild and regenerate the strongest weapon you have against illness and aging. Your immune system.

What Is The Immune System

The immune system is an umbrella term referring to the body's ability to protect itself against infection, made possible by the presence of circulating antibodies and white blood cells. Antibodies are manufactured specifically to defuse and knock out infectious threats to your health. White blood cells or phagocytes are needed to devour and destroy harmful substances such as a threatening virus.

Active immunity arises when your body's own cells produce, and remain able to produce, appropriate antibodies following an attack of a disease.

How Your Immune System Offers Protection

For example, if either skin or mucous membrane is damaged, any bacteria can get through. Once these microbes enter, they multiply. Your body must see to it that they do not establish a foothold or multiply beyond control. Your immune system calls upon resistance in the form of antibodies which are formed by your own tissues through nutritional therapy. These same nourished antibodies help to put the microbes out of action. Your immune system then gathers phagocytes or mobile white blood cells. They engulf any harmful bacteria or microbes in their pathway and usually destroy them. This is the basis of your immune system. It is more than just healing—it is lifesaving!

Threats to Your Immune System

Many different substances are capable of threatening the health and vitality of your immune system. These include bacteria, viruses, drugs, pollens, insect venoms, chemicals, climate, and the environment, to name just a few. *Examples:* A winter sniffle can develop into a life-threatening case of the flu that cannot be resisted by a weak immune system. Any common respiratory ailment or allergy could break down your immune system and threaten your life. The list goes on.

Resist Dangers with Nutritional Therapy

Volatile substances can play havoc with your cellular network, break down delicate tissues, upset your body balance, and open the doorway to serious illness. In other words, bacteria run wild can break down your immune system until you have little or no resistance and succumb to the infection. To help you resist such dangers, it is essential to strengthen your fortress of immunity against infection. With the use of specific food groups, the nutrients can act as barriers to protect against penetration or invasion of life-threatening viral bacteria.

How to Feed Yourself a Strong Immune System

With the use of these food groups, you will be able to activate and energize your built-in protectors to help resist these threats to your health. Some of the most potential nutritional immune builders available include the following:

Vitamin A

Vital for influencing the activity of your immune system. It increases the size of the thymus, a special fist-sized lymph gland behind the breastbone that produces many active "defense cells" and other protective T-lymphocytes or disease-fighting substances. These cells may actually be your body's first line of defense against illnesses including cancer.

One of vitamin A's key roles involves cell differentiation. This nutrient helps special cells "recognize" or alert themselves to begin producing specific protein or antibodies needed to combat a particularly threatening microorganism. Vitamin A helps your immune system to detect sooner and respond faster to viral invaders.

Helps Soothe Viral Stress. If infectious bacteria strike, your body is subjected to a form of stress that leads to increased breakdown of body tissue, weight loss as well as a suppressed immune system. To counteract, vitamin A is able to *reduce* symptoms of stress, then enlarge your thymus gland which is otherwise shrunk by stress. This gives you the edge or advantage in decreasing toxicity of the bacterial invasion and helping to fight back and overcome viral stress. Vitamin A liberates your immune system so it rises up and knocks out the infectious threat to your health and life.

Nutritional Sources of Vitamin A: Consider sweet potatoes, corn on the cob, whole or skim milk, carrots, squash, broccoli, asparagus, tomato, cantaloupe, mangoes, apricots, and liver (beef, veal, or chicken). The liver group is also high in fat and cholesterol. You would help boost your immune system with a balanced daily intake of the other meatless sources of vitamin A. A moderate portion of liver just one day a week should help to give you much needed protection against immune system breakdown.

Vitamin Beta-Carotene

It is converted into vitamin A and is needed to improve the secretion of mucus, tears, and saliva. It is especially necessary for the maintenance of the structure of tiny organelles inside the epithelial cells, called secretory vesicles. These cells have specialized functions relating to the protection of your vital organs and the secretion of special fluids. It has been cited as a potent fighter of cancer cells and is highly recommended as a means of building immunity to the ravages of this disease.

Nutritional Sources of Beta-carotene: This is the orange-colored pigment found in foods such as carrots and cantaloupe. In particular, look for the yellow or orange pigment found in melons, squash, apricots, peaches, and carrots. These nutrients are also found in green leafy vegetagbles, although their color is masked by the green pigment chlorophyll.

Vitamin C

This water-soluble nutrient beefs up your immune system. It strengthens your lymphocytes to fight infection. This battle uses up the nutrient, so a fresh supply must always be available if you expect your immune system to be the winner and keep you alive and well. Vitamin C helps to pep up the metabolism of specific lymphocytes, making them react faster and stronger. Vitamin C also increases the number of what are known as receptor sites on a lymphocyte's membrane, making it easier for the lymphocyte to latch on to a dangerous bacteria or virus and destroy this threat.

A unique function is that vitamin C on a daily basis will significantly increase the blood levels of interferon and reduce risk of illness. Interferon is produced by a cell that has been invaded by a virus. It induces surrounding cells to produce proteins to act as a barrier of protection against the virus.

Vitamin C has still more important immune-fighting powers. It is used for the growth and health of the connective tissues in your bodies known as collagen. This cementlike material holds your body together. It can also wrap cancerous tumors in a tough skin of fibrous tissue, encapsulating them, preventing their spreads. It is vitamin C that prompts the proliferation of these connective tissue fibers to surround dangerous viral and other infectious threats.

Nutritional Sources of Vitamin C: Enjoy fruits such as the guava, strawberries, papaya, orange, cantaloupe, honeydew, gooseberries, grapefruit, and tangerines. Vegetables include turnip greens, peppers (green or red), kale, broccoli, Brussels sprouts, cauliflower, cabbage, tomatoes, and potatoes. *Caution:* Cooking drains out the water-soluble vitamin C so plan to eat fruits and vegetables and their juices in a raw state. The potato should be cooked, of course, in a covered kettle to minimize losses.

Vitamin B-Complex

While all members of this family work together, several stand out as being leaders in the war against infection. Vitamin B_6 (pyridoxine), pantothenic acid, and folate are needed to stimulate cellular (T and B cells) and humoral (antibody production) immunity. These three vitamins stimulate antibody-producing cells and strengthen their ability to produce special proteins (immunoglobulins) that fight off foreign invaders. These vitamins nourish the tissues that produce lymphocytes, increase white blood cell numbers, and bestow more youthful immunity. So we see these nutrients are vital performers in their roles of cellular metabolism and boosting immunity.

Nutritional Sources of Vitamin B-Complex. Utilize whole grain breads and cereals, soybeans, legumes, brewer's yeast, asparagus, beets, broccoli, Brussels sprouts, cantaloupes, grapefruit, oranges, and strawberries.

Zinc

This mineral nourishes your immune-building thymus gland. It is zinc that stimulates your thymus to release a hormone, called FTS, which is intimately involved in granting immunity. Zinc is essential for the release of thymic hormones. These, in turn, build T-cells, or types of lymphocytes crucial to the fight against viral and bacterial infections. Zinc also increases the activity of protective lymphocytes that are able to destroy a virus- or bacteria-invaded cell. These lymphocytes are considered part of your body's first line of defense against illness. Zinc is needed to heal the skin and internal mucous membranes.

Nutritional Sources of Zinc: Enjoy wheat germ, wheat bran, brown rice, whole grain breads and cereals, cowpeas (blackeye), skim milk, and cheddar cheese.

Iron

Long known for helping to ward off infections, this mineral is a powerhouse in stimulating your immune system. Basically, the phagocytes, or white blood cells that serve as your body's primary defense mechanism against bacterial infections, depend on iron-containing enzymes to function. These phagocytes engulf bacteria and secrete a variety of corrosive substances known as oxidants, which digest the invading microbe once it is engulfed. Phagocytes need plenty of oxygen to produce cleansing peroxides and depend on iron to bring these substances to them.

Other white blood cells, such as the lymphocytes, function adequately only in the presence of iron. Lymphocytes need iron for energy metabolism and for the production of enzymes important to their very specialized roles in the immune response. The production of protective antibodies also requires iron-dependent enzymes. To strengthen your front line of major defense against viral infections, nourish your body with immune-building iron.

Nutritional Sources of Iron: Enjoy whole grain breads and cereals, wheat bran, brewer's yeast, soybeans, legumes, green peas, Brussels sprouts, chard, prunes and prune juice, and liver (high in fat and cholesterol, so eat sparingly).

The science of immunology has long known there is a connection between immunity and nutrition. It is not that *certain* nutrients affect the immune system. It's that *every* nutrient affects the immune system. By using nutritional therapy with everyday foods, you help to put more vigor and health into your body and mind, via the nourished immune system.

The Immune-Building Power of Garlic

This volatile vegetable is a powerhouse of immune-building factors that will help to protect you against common and uncommon disorders. In particular, it has been said that garlic gives forth a strange type of ultraviolet radiation, called mitogenetic radiations. They have the power of stimulating cell growth and activity. They have a rejuvenative effect on nearly all body functions.

Garlic increases DNA-RNA or genetic code levels, which simultaneously inhibit bacterial spread and viral infection. Garlic also has substances known as *allistatin* that are able to protect against problems of chronic colitis, gastritis, winter ailments, and disorders of the respiratory tract.

Garlic is also a prime source of *germanium,* a trace mineral, that is able to protect against cellular disorders such as found in cancer. Garlic, with this mineral, helps to build and regenerate your entire immune system.

Helps to Detoxify Your System. Garlic is a powerful detoxifier. It neutralizes toxins present in the digestive tract. It cleanses the eliminative organs and enriches the bloodstream. It improves the health of your liver, kidneys, nervous system, and circulatory system. Garlic, an antitoxin, strengthens your resistance against allergens. In brief, garlic neutralizes body pollution be it from man-made chemicals such as food additives, preservative, artificial colorings, or chemical pesticides, or from various poisons and toxic accumulations from the environment.

Garlic may well be the most single powerful food that will help to build your resistance against disease or ailments of the immune system.

Just two or three cloves of garlic daily, chewed raw, diced into a salad, or added to a soup or stew or casserole or blenderized in a vegetable juice, will give a "shot" to your immune system and boost your health.

RESISTS INFECTIONS, DEVELOPS IMMUNITY TO RESPIRATORY DISORDERS WITH NUTRITIONAL THERAPY

Oscar B. was always catching colds; often, he was wheezing and coughing and gasping for air if he was exposed to the slightest cold air. He had a noticeable weakness in his immune system. He was dangerously sensitive to any virus going around. He would become bedridden for days, even weeks. Recovery was very slow.

His immunologist suggested he fortify his diet with vitamins and minerals from foods listed above. He was also told to have three garlic cloves daily, in any form. Oscar B. was anxious to try any therapy that offered hope for strengthening his inner fortress of immunity.

Within nine days, he not only cured his current respiratory attack, but was so alert and strong, he could go in all kinds of weather with nary any attack. He no longer was an "instant invalid" because of the immune-building nutritional foods. Rather, he was "instant immune" and in top-notch health!

Instant Immune-Building Morning Tonic

Combine 1 tablespoon brewer's yeast with 2 scrubbed and cut carrots, sun-dried apricots, citrus fruit wedges, 2 tablespoons wheat germ, 3 garlic cloves, and 6 ounces of salt-free vegetable juice. Blenderize for 3 minutes. When thoroughly combined, drink slowly in the morning.

Benefits: The rich concentration of vitamin A, beta-carotene, vitamin C, zinc and iron, and other trace elements, with the superpower of garlic are thoroughly blended. Within moments, they help to flood your immune system with the power to manufacture needed red and white blood cells to guard against infectious bacteria. In the morning, without interference of competing foods, these nutrients work swiftly to give you a "shot in the arm" and total protection against nutritionally deficient weaknesses. It is like having "instant immunity" in the morning for the rest of the day, and then some.

STRENGTHENS IMMUNE SYSTEM WITH NUTRIENT-PACKED TONIC

Sophie O. complained of constant weakness, sharp weight fluctuations, and digestive upset. The slightest change in weather would leave her coughing, weak, and exhausted before noontime. She was diagnosed as having a nutritionally deficient immune system. Her internist recommended the Instant Immune-Building Morning Tonic. From the very first day, she experienced a rebound. Sophie O. was stronger, could maintain her weight, had no digestive troubles, and could breathe and work with youthful vitality. She takes this tonic every morning and now boasts "the strongest immune system in town!"

Nutrition Helps to Improve Total Health

The defensive and reparative processes are complex functions, involving many different cells, tissues, organs, and systems. Nutrients are interwoven with most of these functions. If one link in the chain is weakened, the result might fall short of expectations, even though all other aspects of the process are intact. It is important to use all elements of nutrition as a connected chain link to enjoy the rewards of total health. It begins with your immune system. Nourish this lifesaving inner fortress, and you will enjoy the best of everything, in body and mind.

HIGHLIGHTS

1. Feed yourself a strong immune system with the use of selected nutrients.
2. Vitamin A, beta-carotene, vitamin C, vitamin B-complex, zinc, and iron are able nutritionally to bolster the protective powers of your immune system. These nutrients are found in everyday foods.
3. Garlic is able to build immune power because of its unique detoxifying substances and elements not easily found in most foods.
4. Oscar B. corrected respiratory weakness by using the important foods to help make him "instant immune."
5. Sophie O. strengthened her system with the Instant Immune-Building Morning Tonic.

——— 20 ———

How to Stay "Forever Young" with Nutritional Therapy

You may notice a strand or two of gray hair, but the newer knowledge of the science of nutritional therapy indicates that many signs of aging can be prevented or at least postponed with the proper foods. Specific nutrients are able to activate sluggish glands, stimulate the immune system, and repair biological assaults to help rebuild and regenerate your body and mind to help you enjoy perpetual youth. By getting to the root cause of aging and correcting it with nutritional therapy, you can stay young longer.

Free Radicals—The Real Cause of Aging

Research into the aging process has recently discovered that the aging process is linked to unstable chemical fragments called *free radicals*. Produced in the body during metabolism, they are short-lived but destructive. They are capable of damaging body tissues, especially cell membranes. Free radicals are molecules which have unstable electrical charges. They are highly reactive with other nearby molecules.

During the oxidative process, free radicals attack lipids (fats) to form compounds called aldehydes and other oxidative by-products, which react with proteins and generate cross-linked aggregates. These fragments circulate throughout the system. They enter the cell membranes to cause injury. Inside the cell are mitochondria, which look like little pillows; inside the mitochondria, are two little membranes called *cristae*. These are the membranes assaulted by free radical reactions.

241

Danger from Damage to Cells

Once a free radical reaction starts in any of these sites, there will be a propagating reaction that will rapidly expand itself and produce very severe injury. Your cells, organs, and systems start to deteriorate. It is a slow process that can begin in your early twenties when the aging process takes root. Reactions can be seen and felt on a gradual basis.

You Can Detect Premature Aging

Look for signs of skin sag; loss of muscle tone; sensitivity to air, light, and heat; constant respiratory disorders; and vital organ weakness. One biological age marker is lipofuscin or age pigment. The influence of free radicals is to make more and more lipofuscin until it saturates every tissue of the body to induce unwanted and undesirable aging. These are just some of the reactions of the free radicals or mischief makers in your system. They are the root causes of aging.

Nutritional Antioxidants Build
Immunity to Free Radicals

A group of nutrients, identified as antioxidants, can bolster your immune response so that you resist the onslaught of the free radicals. These antioxidants may be called *scavengers,* as they sweep through the system, gather up the corrosive fragments and roots, and wash them out of the system. These nutritional antioxidants slow up the accumulation of lipofuscin, a by-product of free radical damage. They defuse these roots, take the power out of their destructive bent, and help to protect your body against unwarranted aging.

How Antioxidants Promote Youthfulness

When oxygen combines with substances such as fats, they turn rancid. This gives rise to the formation of free radicals. Antioxidants tend to control or block this rancidity. They serve as nutritional preservatives. They regulate the oxidative risk to maintain a form of internal purity. Your cells stay younger longer, and so do you!

Example: Place a small piece of raw meat on a plate. Let it remain at room temperature for several days, perhaps less. It starts to spoil, turn rancid, or just plain rot away! You can see the ravages of the oxidative process. The meat fat plus oxygen caused the spoilage because of the exposure to free radicals. The same happens within your molecular structure when fats and oxygen combine during the normal metabolic process.

You cannot avoid fats, nor should you, because they are found in almost every type of food. But you can build resistance to spoilage with the use of antioxidants. You can immunize your body against free-radical aging with nutritional therapy.

How Antioxidants Rescue You from Aging

You want to maintain health and youth by protecting your cell membrane or lining from oxidation. The reason is that oxidation pits and corrodes the cell membrane similar to the way in which it causes rust to form on iron. Oxidation makes it easier for dangerous bacteria and harmful viruses to enter the cell, cause chromosome damage, and lead to cell death or mutation (which could cause cancer.)

New research theorizes that your vulnerability to various age-related disorders such as arthritis, cancer, and certain infections stem from free-radical damage to lymphocytes (white blood cells) that help your immune systems fight off viruses and other infectious agents.

Danger: Oxidation can be caused by free radicals. These tiny molecular particles, compounds containing unpaired, highly charged electrons, are very unstable. They are troublemakers. They literally seize the electrons of other molecules and claim them as their own. *Risk:* They combine with fatty acids to form peroxides, which are caustic to cell membranes. A chain reaction creates more free radicals. This same chain reaction may be a cause of autoimmune diseases, in which the lymphocytes attack the body's own tissues.

Antioxidants work by helping to foil free-radical destruction of cell membranes. These nutritional therapeutic lifesavers protect body cells against unwanted reactions with oxygen but allow the desirable oxygen reactions to proceed without interference. They act as nutritional guardians to keep the oxidative process under strict and safe control.

Source of Lifesaving, Life-Extending Antioxidants

These cell protectors are found in a group of nutrients that put a damper on the power of harmful free radicals. They include the following:

Vitamin A

This nutrient helps to suppress the malignancy of cultured cells transformed by radiation, chemicals, or viruses. It helps to delay the development of free radicals and will also boost immunity. Vitamin A strengthens the epithelial cells (lining body cavities such as mouth, lungs, throat, stomach, intestines, skin, even retina of the eyes), to protect against invasion of harmful viruses. Vitamin A is released form storage depots in the liver to help cells combat the action of the free radicals.

Beta-carotene

It is partially converted into vitamin A for use in strengthening your system. Solely from vegetable or fruit sources, some beta-carotene is *not* converted but becomes involved in maintaining the structure of tiny organelles inside your epithelial cells, or secretory vesicles. Beta-carotene helps to protect your cells against toxicity.

Vitamin C

A water-soluble nutrient, its potent antioxidizing effect takes place *inside* the cell, in the watery fluid. When vitamin C soaks up free radicals, it forms two lifesaving compounds, dehydroascrobic acid and 2,3-diketogulonic acid that is believed to have cancer-fighting properties. Vitamin C also beefs up your immune system by using stronger lymphocytes to fight infection. This antioxidant is needed for the growth and health of collagen, the connective tissue that holds your body together. Vitamin C also blocks the cancer-promoting effects of nitrosamines. There is some evidence that it suppresses the growth of human leukemia cells in culture. Disease- and age-fighting white blood cells are partly dependent upon this nutrient. It boosts the production and activity of interferon, a virus-fighting substance produced by the body.

Vitamin E

Its major function is to act as a scavenger, absorbing the dangerous oxidative by-products and sweeping them out of the body. It is involved in the DNA-RNA process which regulates health and aging. It helps to strengthen the immune barrier, protecting against cross-linkage of cells and organ systems. Vitamin E protects against harmful by-products believed to be involved in the breakdown of the immune system. Vitamin E is believed to protect against excessive production of lipofuscin, the biological age marker. By minimizing the deleterious free-radical reactions, there is hope for freedom from aging and age-related disease.

Selenium

This trace mineral appears to be a potent immune system stimulator. It boosts antibody production. It strengthens resistance to lysosome damage in which free radicals actually rupture membranes, causing a spillage and subsequent destruction of other tissues. Selenium will also control accumulation of lipofuscin (age pigment) which interferes with cellular health and rejuvenation. It protects cells from mutagenic peroxides and breaks down lipid (fat) peroxides that can contribute to arterosclerosis. Thus, selenium is a key component of the body's defense against accelerated aging.

Zinc

A potent antioxidant in that it is an immunity booster. Zinc is needed for the body to make protein. Zinc-containing enzymes help to string together the long chains of amino acids that make up each protein molecule. Every cell's genetic material, its DNA-RNA, is derived from protein. This means that your body must have zinc to make every one of its cells, from the hair on your head to the soles of your feet. Zinc helps to build your immune system to resist aging. Zinc is needed for the massive buildup of infection-fighting white blood cells. Zinc is also required for the uptake of vitamin A by the epithelial cells. This antioxidant mineral appears to interact with vitamin A, a nutrient believed to have an important protective effect against cancer. Its important purpose is to convert free radicals called hydroperoxides into less damaging alcohols that can be speedily eliminated.

Had Your Antioxidants Today?

Boost your resistance to the destructive free radicals with the important antioxidants. Include foods from these nutrients (sources appear throughout this book) on a daily basis and watch yourself stay young longer.

REVERSES AGING PROCESS WITH ANTIOXIDANT THERAPY

She insisted she was "too young" for arteriosclerosis, but at age 44, Marie M. did have fatty deposits and also started to show sagging skin, weak resistance to colds, and a general defect in her immune system. She almost sobbed to her reflection that she was getting "old before my time." Her nutritional practitioner and geriatric physician suggested she boost her antioxidants. Tests showed she was deficient in those nutrients needed to protect against aging. Marie M. increased foods rich in antioxidant nutrients. Within five days, an examination showed a welcome lowering of fatty deposits; her skin firmed up, and she up filled with more youthful energy. The antioxidants had given her a new lease on life, reversed the aging process, made her look and feel the picture of health. She could resist many common and uncommon disorders.

The Gland That Keeps You "Forever Young"

New scientific research suggests that the little-known thymus gland may well hold the key to rejuvenation. This is a flat, pinkish-gray, two-lobed gland that nestles behind the sternum and lungs high in your chest. The thymus distributes and nourishes (with its hormones) white blood cells, called lymphocytes, that act as your body's defense against illness.

How Thymus Protects Against Aging

This gland is the headquarters for a group of cells known as T-lymphocytes. When they meet an antagonist such as a free radical, a virus or even a cancer cell, these T-cells are stimulated to divide into larger, active cells that challenge the invader and kill it. T-lymphocyte cells actually gobble up harmful cells and wash them out of your system. Age-causing fragments are knocked out and eliminated. Much of antiaging is involved with an active, protective thymus gland.

Problem: The thymus is at its maximum size during the adolescent years; then it shrinks markedly, reducing the supply of thymic hormones and important T-cells. The aged T-cells decline in their ability to reproduce and stimulate formation of antibodies. This can bring on aging as well as a weakened control of the immune system. *Danger:* The shrinking of the thymus and simultaneous decline in T-cell function may be responsible for premature aging and increasing illness among folks in their thirties and forties, even younger. These were once thought to be part of the inevitable so-called aging process. But newer knowledge of nutrition holds that the thymus can be nutritionally strengthened, even though smaller in size, to protect against debilitation and aging.

Nutritional Therapy Invigorates Thymus

This gland releases thymosin, a hormone that helps to build immunity and resistance against aging. The thymus is a storehouse of zinc, the antioxidant mineral essential to both protein synthesis and cell division. The efficient working of the immune system depends on the rapid proliferation of T-cells; it is zinc that stimulates the thymus to release the hormone to make these age-preventing cells.

Zinc stimulates production of adequate amounts of thymosin which manufactures lymphocytes that cleanse such damaging elements as free radicals that are a threat to your health. Zinc, as a nutritional therapeutic mineral, stimulates your thymus to release thymosin, which, in turn, activates T-lymphocytes to do battle against age-causing threats.

Small but Powerful Nutrient

Your needs of zinc are small but inescapable. A general rule of thumb would be about 15 milligrams per day—to keep aging away! (Food sources of zinc are given throughout this book.)

You *can* extend your prime of life. The young and vigorous science of gerontology is fast homing in on the real reason of aging. The youth searchers have found that one major biological cause is that of nutrition. With the use of proper therapies, the aspect of aging can be halted, or at least many consequences of the process can be prevented or postponed. With nutritional therapy, aging may be abolished!

To put it personally, if you were told there is a way to add productive years to your life while being spared the distress of preventable illness, would you be interested? And would you pursue it even though you knew to attain this goal required a change in your life-style, a new nutritional dedication, and a genuine personal involvement?

The choice is yours.

SUMMARY

1. Aging is largely caused by the mischief-making free radicals circulating throughout your system.

2. Antioxidants are nutrients that knock out and eliminate the damaging free radicals.

3. Rejuvenating antioxidants include vitamin A, beta-carotene, vitamin C, vitamin E, selenium, and zinc that are potent in defusing free

radicals and stimulating your immune system to protect against aging.

4. Marie M. corrected her premature and unwarranted arteriosclerosis, sagging skin, and respiratory weakness with the use of antioxidant nutrients.

5. Your thymus gland needs zinc to release a hormone that helps you stay "forever young."

Index